Healing with
God's Love

Healing with God's Love

Kabbalah's Hidden Secrets

Rabbi Douglas Goldhamer, Ph.D., D.D.

with Peggy Bagley

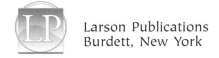

Larson Publications
Burdett, New York

ISBN-10: 1-936012-74-X
ISBN-13: 978-1-936012-74-9
eISBN-10: 1-936012-75-8
eISBN-13: 978-1-936012-75-6

Library of Congress Control Number: 2014951072

Publisher's Cataloging-In-Publication Data
(Prepared by The Donohue Group, Inc.)

Goldhamer, Douglas Hirsch.
   Healing with God's love : Kabbalah's hidden secrets / Rabbi Douglas Goldhamer, Ph.D., D.D., with Peggy Bagley.

     pages ; cm

   Issued also as an ebook.
   Includes bibliographical references and index.
   ISBN-13: 978-1-936012-74-9
   ISBN-10: 1-936012-74-X

   1. Spiritual healing--Judaism. 2. Cabala. 3. Judaism--Prayers and devotions.
4. Mysticism--Health aspects. 5. Meditation--Therapeutic use. 6. Visualization--
Therapeutic use. I. Bagley, Peggy. II. Title.

BM729.H43 G65 2015
296.76   2014951072

Published by Larson Publications
4936 State Route 414
Burdett, New York 14818 USA

https://www.larsonpublications.com

24 23 22 21 3019 18 17 16 15
10 9 8 7 6 5 4 3 2 1

We dedicate this book to our
beloved teachers and mentors,
Rabbi Dr. Yaakov Dresher, z"l, and
Rabbi Daniel Dresher, z"l.
It would not exist without their
knowledge, kindness, and skills.

Contents

God's Healing Prayer—
Exodus 15:26

"He said, if you will heed the Lord your God diligently, doing what is upright in His sight, giving ear to His commandments and keeping all His laws, then I will not bring upon you any of the diseases . . ."

I became interested in the Jewish model of healing when I realized that no doctors could help me with my disease of Klippel-Trenaunay syndrome, a debilitating vascular disorder which impeded my ability to walk. My doctors said that both my legs needed to be amputated. I was devastated by this diagnosis, but because of my strong faith, I knew that God would not abandon me. I turned even more deeply to my faith and learned of a Jewish healer, Rabbi Daniel Dresher.

I will always remember when Rabbi Dresher first told me there are healing mysteries in the Bible. He said I could obtain healing through prayer, that healing is Biblical. I was amazed when I turned to Exodus 15:26 and read: "He [God] said, if you will heed the Lord your God diligently, doing what is upright in His sight, giving ear to His commandments and keeping all His laws, then I will not bring upon you any of the diseases . . ."[1] Rabbi Dresher and, later, his nephew Rabbi Dr. Yaakov Dresher directed me to Hebrew texts with amazing, holy, meaningful, and highly effective insights for healing.

Rabbi Daniel Dresher died many years ago, and Rabbi Dr. Yaakov Dresher, z"l,[2] passed away in April of 2013. He was my mentor and very dear friend. It was he who really showed me, through texts and the example of his practice, that Jewish healing practice has an enormous moral component. It is beyond moral. It is all about God.

As Melinda Stengel and I discussed in our book *This Is for Everyone,* and Peggy and I will show in more depth here, the letters of the Hebrew alphabet are very powerful. When we invoke their energies for healing, it is essential to do so with good motivation and in the right spirit. The more understanding we have of God's nature and our relationships with it, the better suited we are to heal.

Jewish tradition gives us many names through which to approach understanding God's nature. Many of them address God's transcendent or "masculine" qualities. *YHVH,* for example, pronounced *Yod Hey Vav Hey* and written in Hebrew as יהוה,[3] is a name for the transcendent or masculine aspect of God. The sequence of letters *Yod Hey Vav Hey* is energetically so strong and powerful that Kabbalists call *YHVH* the Face of God or *Tetragrammaton.*

When the Lord first revealed this name to Moses through the burning bush in Exodus, Ch. 6, He also revealed that prior to this holy encounter between them, God had appeared to the patriarchs in feminine form as *El Shaddai,* which translates as God of Breasts. God appeared to the matriarchs and patriarchs, as told in the Book of Genesis, as a nurturing deity expressing feminine qualities. God now relates to Moses that, in the future, we must also recognize God's masculine Name, the God who governs the universe, the God of history.

El Shaddai corresponds to the immanent nature of God, Her Feminine Presence. God's immanent Feminine Presence is also called *Shechina.* Through the *Shechina* we gain direct experience of the transcendent deity, and through the *Shechina,* healing takes place. Embrace *YHVH* by embracing the sacred Feminine, and none of the diseases that plague the world will hurt you.

Healing begins when we embrace this awareness of unity. When we see ourselves as separate from God, we are prone to illness. But when we know that God is in everything and that we need to repair the unity of all things in God, we are on the road to wellness. When we recognize that each of us is divine because each of us is part of God, we are on the way to complete healing.

When the Romans destroyed the Jewish temple in 70 AD and exiled the people of Israel, the *Shechina*, the Feminine Presence of God or God's indwelling Presence in Creation, went into exile with them. Because of Her enormous compassion and love for them, She exiled Herself from Her male consort and there was a metaphorical split in the Divine. The transcendent male aspect of God, *YHVH*, also known as *HaKodesh Barchu, The Holy One, blessed be He*, continued to govern the universe, and God's feminine nature, the *Shechina* or Indwelling Presence, went into exile with the Jewish people.[4]

Rabbi Shneur Zalman of Liadi (1745–1812) explains the exile of the *Shechina* in his magnum opus *Tanya, Igeret HaKodesh* 31. In this work, he elaborates on how the Kabbalah views the causes of illness. We learn that, just as illness is a result of our false belief that we are separate from God, illness also is the result of the *Shechina's* suffering in Her exile and in Her separation from Her male consort. Unity, our belief in the unification of everything in God, leads to healing. Separation, our belief that we are all separate beings and that the *Shechina* is separate from *YHVH*, leads to illness and disease.

The cause of the destruction of the ancient temple was "baseless hatred" of Jew against Jew during those times. This caused the temple to be destroyed, the exile to take place, and the Feminine Presence of God to separate from *YHVH*. I further believe that the metaphorical split in the Divine, with illness and disease as a result, was caused and continues to be caused by hate in this world — not only hate by Jews against fellow Jews, but hate for all people by all people. Only true love brings about healing and wellness. This true love needs to be predicated on the idea that everything and everyone is made up of the stuff we call God.

Love is the antidote that will bring about healing. Love is the life-giving blood that unites us and God. We need to focus on the *Shechina* and alleviate Her suffering by bringing Her out of Her exile.

Love — true love — brings unity, the recognition that we are all one and one in God. "All" here applies equally to Jews and non-Jews. We need to undo the exile that is based on separateness, and we need to bring together, through love, the unity of God in everyone and everything.

This is a profound secret of Kabbalistic healing: Not only is it through the *Shechina* that we gain direct experience of the transcendent Deity, but it is through our embracing of the *Shechina* that healing takes place. The Feminine aspect of God plays a most important role in healing.

Throughout this book we show in different ways how, when we elevate the *Shechina* and when we recognize the importance of *YHVH*'s *Shechina* in our prayers, we will achieve healing. This is a very important theme that I constantly embrace when I do healing with my parishioners. The results are extraordinary.

Remember: When you pray for healing, you are to pray for the *Shechina*, for God's Indwelling Presence. It is said that She is the aspect of God that is intimately connected with all the souls of Israel. She is also called the "Community of Israel," a way the ancients tried to make their contemporaries aware that all Jewish souls were bound together as one single soul.

Such was the thinking of the originators and creators of the early Kabbalah, and even the writers of the later Kabbalah of the Middle Ages. They wrote this way to give the Jewish community hope for survival in the face of the great tragedy of the Roman destruction of the ancient temple in 70 AD and the equal tragedy of the Jewish massacre and expulsion from Spain in the fifteenth century — to give the Jewish people of their times a theology of hope.

I believe that if these same Kabbalists and rabbis were alive today, they would recognize that the Feminine Presence of God is in all people, not only Jewish people. Conditions today, with suffering in Rwanda, Syria, Israel, and throughout the world, require us to recognize that the Presence of God dwells within each one of us, regardless of ethnicity or personal religious upbringing. I believe that the thinking of the ancient rabbis was right on the mark for that time, and that thinking on this point has evolved.

We now can understand, thanks to their amazing insights, that God does not live in the heavens alone, nor does She live only in the souls of Jews. She lives within all of us and loves all of us. This awareness allows us to realize that She is One, and that when we pray for Her healing, we pray for everyone's healing. The child who suffers heart disease in Syria, the child who suffers heart disease in Austria, and the child who suffers heart disease in a Birmingham hospital — when we pray for the healing of the *Shechina* who lives in all these children, we are also praying for our own child with heart disease. This was the amazing realization of the thinkers of the Kabbalah.

If you understand how we are all connected, and if you focus on how the *Shechina* suffers together with all those who suffer, if you identify your personal pain with Hers, you are no longer alone. When you pray for others as well as yourself, knowing you are no longer alone, you become a direct conduit of healing for yourself and others.

When you pray for the diminution of your own disease, you need to pray not only for yourself; you need to pray for the well-being of others with this same disease. You must pray with great passion for their well-being. When you pray this way, you will be privy to a great secret of healing. You become a vessel drawing in divine light for yourself and those around you. You draw down the Transcendent Light of *YHVH*, lift up the *Shechina* Light — *Adonai ADNY* אדני — and allow healing to take place.

There are other Kabbalistic healing insights that we learn from Exodus 15:26. First, illness is connected to ethical action: There is an ethical basis to health and illness, and a direct correlation between the human healer and the Divine healer. God is clearly teaching us that if we want to escape disease, we need to practice ethical precepts. We need to be good.

Righteous behavior allows us to bring the Divine energies in every cell into balance. The unhealthy person's cells are out of balance, weighed down by *Shechina* energy only. Ethical behavior with *kavvanah* meditation lifts up the *Shechina* and joins Her with the aspect of the Divine that brings good health and balanced Divine energies into every cell.

This great secret teaches that there is an ethical and moral basis for health. It is important to obey the Ten Commandments and other *mitzvoth* (plural of *mitzvah*) commandments, conscious connections, actions in harmony with the Higher Mind. *Jewish medicine, distinct from the medical model taught at American universities, is completely related to moral, ethical, and spiritual values.* Kabbalah teaches that it is not enough to repair a broken arm or treat a cancer with sophisticated chemotherapy: If we want real healing, it is crucial to bring in the moral context of a person's illness. There is more to illness and healing than meets the eye.

We reveal many secrets about correlations between health and morality in this book. If we don't mention moral practice in a specific meditation, remember always that it is essential for you to love the person you are praying for, love yourself, and love God. You need to actually *feel* love and compassion during your healing meditative practices. Without love, all the technical knowledge won't work. For healing to take place, spiritual technology must be joined with love. We can't emphasize enough how important that is.

When we consciously unite the male and female Divine energies, we embrace what the great healing Kabbalists taught again and again — something most often spoken of today as mindfulness. The Kabbalists, in doing their healing, highlighted the importance of embracing the present moment, recognizing the Divinity within this very moment. *This idea of uniting the Male and Female aspects of God is a key principle,* possibly the single most important secret we are trying to teach here.

There is divinity in everything and in every moment. You must not only embrace this idea, you must make it your own. When you recognize the importance of attending to the Divine at every moment, when you consciously recognize that God is not only a He but also manifests the great Feminine Principle, and when you understand that you are given the *mitzvah*, the command, to unite male and female in every holy moment — then you will begin to be an instrument of God who is not only *aware* of healing, but one who actively *promotes* healing. We thank our wonderful teacher Rabbi Dr. Yaakov Dresher, z"l, and our mentor Rabbi Daniel Dresher, z"l, for bringing us to understand this.

In addition to our beloved teachers and mentors to whom we dedicate this book, we want to thank Officers Joel Bemis and Dino Amato, two Chicago cops with whom we have shared wonderful scotch and even more wonderful spiritual and theological discussions. These two guys are the best, and we love them. Jewish tradition shows enormous respect for non-Jews who embrace the principles of virtuous living that we aspire to. We call such people righteous. Joel and Dino are righteous.

We also want to thank Congregation Bene Shalom for their kind support of us. We particularly extend our appreciation to our dear friend Nona Balk, assistant Rabbi Shari Chen, cantorial soloist Charlene Brooks, Ava Eres, and temple president Rita Carroll. All were instrumental in ensuring that the temple continued to run smoothly while we were working on this book. We also would like to thank Granite Amit for all her help and support. Finally, Peggy and I also want to thank Paul Cash, our editor and publisher, for his tremendous faith and support as we brought this project to fruition.

Douglas Goldhamer
Peggy Bagley
October 2014

NOTES

1. Throughout this book, we will use *The Torah: A Modern Commentary* (Union of American Hebrew Congregation, New York, 1981). Commentaries by W. Gunther Plaut.

2. z"l is a contraction from the Hebrew *zichron letov,* which means *May he be remembered for the good*.

3. Readers unfamiliar with Hebrew should note that the letters *YHVH, Yod Hey Vav Hey,* are read from right to left in the Hebrew characters, so that the first *Yod* י is at the right, the first *Hey* ה to its left, the *Vav* ו to the left of that, and the final *Hey* ה all the way to the left: יהוה

4. Another Rabbinic narrative teaches that the *Shechina* left her male consort when God expelled Adam and Eve from the Garden of Eden. Her compassion for Her children was so great that She followed them into exile.

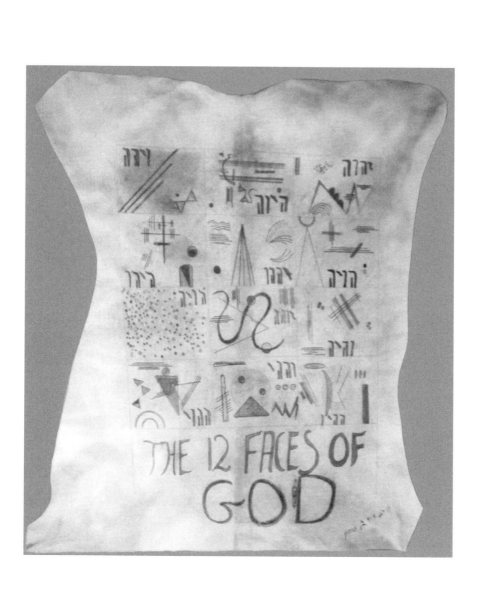

Introduction

Life is full of synchronistic moments.

In 1976 I was diagnosed with Klippel-Trenaunay syndrome, a rare vascular disease. It had caused blood clots in my left leg for many years, forcing me to walk first with a cane and later with crutches.

Before this diagnosis, doctors had been treating me for a propensity for blood clotting by surgically removing not only the clots, but also the veins in which they were located. Several surgeries had left me in excruciating pain. It was only through my own research that I discovered I had been walking around with Klippel-Trenaunay syndrome all my life.

When I showed the surgeons my discovery, they suggested amputation of my left leg, and perhaps my right leg as well. Amputation was a common treatment for Klippel-Trenaunay.

Understandably, I did not want my legs to be amputated. At that time I was dating the girl who would later become my wife. I thought, would she stay with an amputee? I soon realized that I had misjudged her. Peggy is a beautiful angel, and we have now been married for thirty-three years.

As I refused to have my leg amputated, the doctors said they could not help me except by prescribing blood thinners and pain medication. So, I searched for alternative healing. I had graduated from rabbinical school, and felt that I always had a very close friendship with God, which inclined me to be very open to alternative healing. I soon met a mystical rabbi, Rabbi Daniel Dresher, who taught me new ways to meditate and pray. His approach was based on certain ways of using the ancient Hebrew letters, Kabbalistic *kavvanot* or meditative activities, and spiritual healing techniques practiced by ancient Kabbalistic communities.

Rabbi Dresher was a Hasidic teacher with enormous patience and tremendous learning. He welcomed Peggy and me into his home, even though I am not an Orthodox rabbi. It was here that he did Kabbalistic healing with me and shared his vast store of knowledge about healing with us every week.

After almost a year of weekly visits, of learning, praying, and meditating, I was greatly healed. I put away my crutches and canes and began applying these healing techniques with members of my own congregation who were experiencing various diseases. I saw that ancient Hebrew meditative spiritual techniques, combined with Western medical knowledge, could achieve phenomenal results. I shared my newfound insights in a book with Melinda Stengel on Jewish mysticism and the healing arts, entitled *This Is for Everyone.*

Subsequent to my healing and writing that text, I have continued to practice Kabbalistic healing meditations with many members of my community. I have refined old healing methods and studied many more Kabbalistic texts in these intervening years. I continually see that our esoteric Jewish tradition is rich with diverse healing techniques. Furthermore, I have seen the efficacy of these healing *kavvanot* with members of my congregation and even asked some of them to share their remarkable healing experiences with you.

For this book, I have invited Peggy Bagley, my wife and best friend, to collaborate with me. She is a superb writer and, more importantly, an intuitive spiritual practitioner who often prays with me and the people with whom I do healing.

This new book is filled with spiritual techniques and Kabbalistic meditations that we did not discuss in *This Is for Everyone.* I have seen such great success with these healing meditations through the years that I now want to share my discoveries. Peggy and I also go into great depth to explain beautiful Kabbalistic concepts that are the basis and source for these meditations.

After several years of practicing and teaching spiritual healing, I received a telephone call from an old friend. She asked if I could please meet with her sister, who was very ill with a cancer that had metastasized to her liver. I flew to her home city and, through a series of events, met Rabbi Dr. Yaakov Dresher, the nephew of my previous teacher Rabbi Daniel Dresher.

The chances of my meeting Rabbi Yaakov were almost impossible, had not God directed our meeting. In addition to his rabbinical ordination, Rabbi Yaakov chose to pursue a Ph.D. in mathematics. He was thrilled to meet me and talk about his favorite uncle Daniel. He took me under his wing, and directed me to many new Kabbalistic sources. For thirteen years, he taught me Kabbalistic healing meditations and prayers that I had not studied with his uncle. This is why Peggy and I dedicate this book to the Dresher family — Rabbi Daniel Dresher, z"l and Rabbi Dr. Yaakov Dresher, z"l.

If you think that this sounds like a fantastic story, you are right. So let me come clean. I want to share something with you here that I did not share in my first book, for fear then that people would think me crazy. It cannot be a coincidence and happenstance that I met both Rabbis Dresher. What's unusual here is not simply that God is directing my life. Rather, it's what I mean when I now can say that I *see* God directing my life, and that you also can see God directing yours.

It is not so difficult to accept that God is involved in our lives and has a plan for each one of us, even though most of us can't see it. It's another thing to *see* it. Let me tell you how I came to actually see it.

When I wrote *This Is for Everyone,* I shared with no one except my wife Peggy what I share with you now. Yes, Rabbi Dan Dresher taught me and instructed me and prayed with me and directed me to Hebrew Kabbalistic texts, and that was a remarkable experience. But what is even more amazing to me is that I had already learned some of these prayer techniques in a dream, a year before I met him. I understand that this sounds incredible. I myself would have difficulty believing what I am about to say if this hadn't happened to me.

I had just come home from a meeting Peggy and I had with a surgeon at Northwestern Memorial Hospital in Chicago. He said clearly that if I didn't want to die of gangrene poisoning in the future, I would have to have my left leg amputated. I was in a terrible mood and wondered why a good person like myself, who had dedicated his life to teaching Torah in sign language to both deaf and hearing children, would be rewarded with such an ominous decree. I thought the Talmudic rabbi, Rabbi Yossi Ha-Gelili in the Talmud was right: "No good deed goes unpunished."

It was with this in mind that I went to sleep that night. I was so angry at God that I refused to say my bedtime prayers, which include the *Sh'ma*.[1] That night I had what can best be described as a supernatural experience. I had a dream, and in my dream a voice spoke with me, instructing me on how to do the Healing Prayer that I outlined in my first book. When I woke up from the dream, I immediately ran up the stairs to my study in the attic and wrote down as much as I could of the healing prayer that I had experienced in my dream. I regret to say, I put the notes aside for the next six months.

When I later met Rabbi Dan Dresher, and he began instructing me and teaching me mystical meditations, I saw that some of these *kavvanot* prayers were identical to the ones I had received in my dream. I was so amazed when I compared my text and notes to his text and notes that I had an epiphany! They were the same! I knew God was working in my life. Like Jacob, I awoke out of my sleep and felt, as Jacob had said, "Surely God is in this place and as for me, I never knew it" (Genesis 28:16).

The ancients are right. We can find God in our dreams. This is not to say that every dream leads you to the Presence of God. *Au contraire!* I have seen that most of my dreams are the result of a great pizza with all the toppings at 11:30 p.m., or the sortings-out in my mind of a very difficult day at work. But with the aid of meditative techniques, we can dream those heavenly dreams that bring us into the Presence of God or His angels.

One of the pleasures of my ministry is to lead our Sunday morning children's worship service. I learn so much from young children. But there is one principle that seems a bit difficult for them to comprehend — the principle is that God is everywhere. When I ask them, "Where is God?" their first response is always "He is in heaven" rather than "She is everywhere." They wonder, if God is everywhere, why is there sickness in my home? Or why does my Aunt Edith still have cancer? Or why does Bob the bully always get away with teasing me?

Adults also wrestle with this problem intellectually: If God is everywhere, why does slavery still exist in the Sudan? Or in Niger? If God is everywhere, why did Auschwitz happen? How could God allow twenty innocent children to be murdered in Newtown, Connecticut? Closer to home, if God is everywhere, why did my daughter die of a brain tumor?

I think the reason my Sunday school children and many adults have a difficult time comprehending that God is everywhere, is because until we have a real religious experience, this great fact is very difficult to understand. Jacob, for example, knew that God was in Be'er Sheva, his childhood home in the Negev area in southern Israel. His parents Isaac and Rebecca were devout believers and they taught all their sons the importance of embracing God in their lives. So this was "normal" for him. But when Jacob later found God also in a strange place — in the strange dream he had of a ladder with angels going up and down, from earth to heaven and heaven to earth — he was overwhelmed. It was a true religious experience, to find God equally present in that Egyptian desert so far from his home. He formed a strikingly new thought "Surely God is in this place and as for me, I never knew it" (Genesis 28:16).

Jacob realized that God is everywhere. In the dream, God makes it very clear that He is not just another local deity. He says to Jacob: "I am the Lord, the God of Abraham, thy father and the God of Isaac . . ." (Genesis 28:13). And with this revelation comes a renewal of God's promise to be wherever Jacob is: "I will be with you, protecting you wherever you go . . ." (Genesis 28:15). Jacob is so inspired and amazed that he shouts, "This place is the place of God. This is the gate of heaven." He concludes with conviction, "Here is the House of God." Equally, here is the Gate of Heaven, and both are wherever we seek them.

This seems like a simple thought. God is up and down, west, south, east, and west. God is everywhere. And yet, I see that with my Sunday school class, or my teachings at the synagogue, people have a hard time grasping that God is not only in the synagogue sanctuary or church chapel, but everywhere. Each community wants to grab hold of God and monopolize Him and call Him by a specific name which identifies Him as theirs and theirs only. It is hard for people to grasp that the God of the Eskimo is the same God as the God of the Jew, and that the God of the Jew must be equally revered as the God of the Baptist. Because there is only one God and God is everywhere. We need to realize that God is as close to us as the air we breathe.

Indeed, this Life Force that we call God is Breath. The Hebrew word for breath is *Ru'ach*. *Ru'ach* also means spirit, and *Ru'ach HaKodesh* means Holy Spirit or Holy Breath. Another name for *Ru'ach* is life energy. In China it is called chi, and in Japan it is ki or qi. In India, this *Ru'ach* is identified as prana, the Sanskrit word for energy. Eastern thought sees chi pass through different meridians that correspond with various organs of the body. The French philosopher Henri Bergson called this life energy the élan vital. In the second verse of its opening chapter, the Hebrew Bible calls it *Ru'ach Elohim,* the Breath of God.

This Breath is the Source of all life. Our covenant with God allows us to enter into a relationship with the Holy Spirit and receive His breath. And when we know how to become one with God's Breath and receive it rhythmically throughout our body, there is healing. Rabbi Nachman of Breslov wrote in his magnum opus, *Likutei Moharan (Collected Writings of Our Teacher)*, that there is a direct correlation between the Psalms and the Divine Breath. He writes that when a person recites the Psalms with the right focus and intention, the reader's own breath inspires the Divine within the words.

It is generally known among Kabbalists that all life originates from a single source called *Ayn Sof,* the One without End. It is the origin and fountain of all energy. This *Ayn Sof* that we call God is really the Life Force that energizes the whole universe. If we could see the Unseen, we would see the movement of a conscious, compassionate, caring, intelligent Energy that moves from the unseen worlds right down to the physical world. This Energy is filled with consciousness and awareness.

In Judaism, God's Energy travels through the human body and is transformed by unique transformers of Energy which we call *Sefirot*.[2] Eastern thought also sees the energy body as having unique points, which they call chakras. These chakras are whirling energy centers. Some systems count the major chakras as numbering eleven or seven. The chakras control, energize, and are responsible for the proper functioning of different parts and organs of the physical body, including the endocrine glands, which receive energy from some of the major chakras. But, whereas the chakras are seen as spiritual energy centers of the human body, the *Sefirot* are not only energy centers but also energy transformers. The similarity between the two is that each chakra or *Sefira* is related to different organs or limbs.

The Kabbalah teaches that this Energy we call God manifests itself as a dichotomy of positive and negative aspects. These opposites attract and cause life. These opposing fields are explained by the *Sefirot*. The *Sefirot* teach how God's energy flows freely from the *Ayn Sof* into every human and everything that occupies our world. God's energy flows freely from the *Ayn Sof* through us and back to Him.

According to Judaism, Creation is not a static event but a dynamic experience. God continually creates the world in which there is a free flow and exchange of energy within each human, and also from God to humans and humans to God. This free flow is not automatic. For the free flow to take place, we have to learn how to work these *Sefirot* or transformers of energy in God and in ourselves. This involves the use of meditations, *kavvanot*, visualizations, and the imaginative faculty, *ko'ach dimyon*. The meditative practices that we find in numerous Kabbalistic texts encourage the flow of God's Energy and allow us to be filled in the best possible way with His Breath. These visualization and imagery techniques, together with breathing techniques, are what the Kabbalists call *kavvanot*, or meditative activities. These spiritual meditative activities allow the practitioner to work in harmony with the Life Force of God.

Jewish tradition holds that around 1200 BCE there was a huge revelation in which God gave the Torah. The Torah is a holy contract or covenant between the two parties. Kabbalists maintain that an esoteric reading of this covenant reveals secret mystical principles that teach how human beings and God can work together to the benefit of spiritual and physical healing.

There is a continuous and constant relationship between the physical and the spiritual. When we recognize this integral relationship, which occurs at all levels, there is great healing. While *Ru'ach* means breath or wind at the physical level, it can be transformed to another level of experience. The same word can mean Holy Spirit when written as *Ru'ach HaKodesh*. But just writing *Ru'ach HaKodesh* is not enough. The internal dynamic of the person inhaling and exhaling *Ru'ach* is what transforms one's sense of the physicality of the world to a high sense of spiritual presencing. When this transformation takes place, profound healing occurs.

Rabbi Yaakov's teachings emphasized the importance of *Ru'ach* and meditative breathing techniques. His uncle, Rabbi Dan, emphasized visualization; but Rabbi Yaakov, though also embracing and mandating visualization techniques, focused equally on breathing techniques for healing. Rabbi Yaakov said constantly that we must identify physical *Ru'ach* with spiritual *Ru'ach*: They are inseparable. Physical and spiritual realities are always together. He taught that a secret of healing is to understand that Kabbalah is holistic.

One Sunday he took from his bookshelf a very large Hebrew volume, published in Jerusalem. It was the book mentioned above, the *Likutei Moharan* (*Collected Writings of Our Teacher*) by Rabbi Nachman of Breslov. Rabbi Nachman was a mystical rabbi who lived in the late eighteenth and early nineteenth centuries. His *Likutei Moharan* is a multi-volume work that teaches there is a powerful relationship between the body and the soul, which has far-reaching implications for physical healing. If we tend to the soul, and correct the transgressions we make and have made in life, this will lead to physical health. He taught that there are soul counterparts to the organs and limbs of the human body. Rabbi Yaakov showed me, in Rabbi Nachman's text, how *Ru'ach* must be understood both physically and spiritually. If we understand this, there is the reward of healing and good health.

Life depends on breath. And what is breath? It is the exhaling and the inhaling of *Ru'ach*. When a person is completely embracing God, speaking Torah and prayer, that person is exhaling and inhaling *Ru'ach HaKodesh*, the Holy Spirit.

We find in Genesis 1:2, "The *Ru'ach* of God hovered over the face of the waters." That is, when a person studies Torah, which itself is like water, then the *Ru'ach* (Breath) of God which is the *Ru'ach HaKodesh* (Holy Spirit) hovers over and breathes life into that person. It is impossible to live without Torah. And we see in the *Tikkunei Zohar 13*, "Were it not for the *Ru'ach* of the lobes of the lungs, fanning and cooling the heart, its heat would consume the whole body."[3]

Likutei Moharan teaches in this section that there is more than a mere "correlation" between physicality and spirituality. When a person breathes with awareness, there is an actual awareness that one's breath *is* the Holy Breath of God, especially when praying or studying. The physical and the spiritual come together. This *Ru'ach* is none other than the Holy Spirit that one inhales when one breathes words of holiness.

We must maintain a balance between the physical and the spiritual in our lives. Just as we must continue to burn God's flame in our hearts so that we are passionate about becoming one with God, we must recognize that our lungs work in harmony with our heart so that our heart runs smoothly and does not overheat.

The Kabbalah teaches that energy vibrates. And since everything is made up of energy, everything is made up of God. Aspects of reality that we call spiritual, such as angels and spiritual beings, move with faster vibrations. Aspects of reality that are more physical, such as rocks and trees and sky-scrapers, move at much slower vibration rates. The human being is made up of all aspects of reality, and as such is a microcosm of reality. We are made up of *Sefirot* that pulsate very quickly and *Sefirot* that vibrate much less quickly. We are made up of flesh and blood and are also composites of feelings and thoughts and soul. The faster energy vibrates, the closer we are to a state of spirituality. But the slower the vibrations, the more we are experiencing the physical world.

God is in every cell of our body. God is the basic stuff out of which we are all made. Rabbi Yaakov taught me that when our energy increases, our cells vibrate more strongly. Theologically speaking, this is what is meant by activating the Presence of God within us. We do this when we increase our energy, and when our cells vibrate at faster speeds, these cells influence other cells to vibrate similarly. (For more on sympathetic vibration, see Chapter 8.)

Rabbi Yaakov taught that we can learn healing modalities that activate another person's awareness of the Presence of God. When we do this kind of Kabbalistic healing with someone who is ill, we help that person rise into a more spiritual dimension in their consciousness — by inspiring him (or her) to recognize that he can activate the Divine Spirit within him. When he does this, *assisted by Kabbalistic meditative techniques,* he heightens his energy levels to higher and faster vibrations. This illustrates Rabbi Nachman's thesis that there is a direct correlation between the spiritual and physical bodies of every human being.

It is worth briefly mentioning here that a person's malady can be caused by having too much energy or overactive cell vibrational activity in one part of the body. We will discuss this later, as well as other Kabbalistic explanations for the origin and cause of disease. But in general, when a person recognizes that God is everywhere, including within every cell of his body, this recognition will heighten his vibrational cellular activity and that will lead to good health. In this book, Peggy and I teach how to facilitate such healing in oneself and in others.

In the Reform Jewish tradition, we read from the Hebrew Torah every Sabbath. My congregation's synagogue is very blessed to have an old Torah that was rescued along with some others from Nazis who seized them during the Holocaust. When we established our synagogue in 1972, it consisted mostly of deaf people. I wrote a letter to a foundation that had collected these sacred scrolls, asking if our nascent congregation could acquire one of the Torahs. I knew that Hitler had murdered more than ten thousand deaf people only because they were deaf. To my great pleasure, the Westminster Project sent us one, free of charge. We read this Torah regularly on our Sabbath and at bar and bat mitzvahs and Jewish holidays.

When I visited with Rabbi Yaakov, I saw that his community did not *read* from the Torah. During the weekdays and on Sabbaths, they would *chant* from the Torah. Our ancient mystical tradition teaches that a person chanting has the power to influence his cellular vibrations, which has a correlative effect on his physical and spiritual development. Chanting, of course, is also embraced by Buddhist monks, and in the Latin of the Catholic Church, among other religious traditions.

As a Kabbalist, I know that it is not simply chanting that influences the vibrational activity of our cells. Some ancient languages are more rich in vibrations than others. We see this, for instance, with Sanskrit and with Hebrew.

We understand the Hebrew language to be very sacred. According to Jewish tradition, inherent in each letter are electric-like forces that God uses to create the Universe. "For when the world was created, it was the supernal letters that brought into being all the works of the lower world, after their own pattern. Hence, whoever has a knowledge of them, and is observant of them, is beloved. Both on high and below."[4] Jewish tradition maintains that God continually creates day and night.

ל	Lamed *has the sound of l*	א	Alef *silent letter*
מ	Mem *has the sound of m*	ב	Bet/Vet *has the sound of b or v*
נ	Nun *has the sound of n*	ג	Gimel *has the sound of g*
ס	Samech *has the sound of s*	ד	Dalet *has the sound of d*
ע	Ayin *silent letter*	ה	Hey *has the sound of h*
פ	Pey/Fey *has the sound of P or F*	ו	Vav *has the sound of v*
צ	Tzadik *has the sound of tz*	ז	Zayin *has the sound of z*
ק	Kuf *has the sound of k*	ח	Chet *has the sound of ch*
ר	Resh *has the sound of r*	ט	Tet *has the sound of t*
ש	Shin/Sin *has the sound of s or sh*	י	Yod *has the sound of y*
ת	Tav *has the sound of t*	כ	Kaph *has the sound of k or kh*

Not only are these letters sacred, but each of the twenty-two Hebrew letters is a specific energy force. They are what God used in various combinations with one another to create the Universe. We humans can use these Hebrew letters to create on Earth.

We can tap into the forces and energies of the Hebrew letters when we recite our prayers in Hebrew. We can see each of these twenty-two energy forces through its different shapes and feel each one through its different sounds. Most importantly, each letter is rich in vibrations that have enormous power in healing. That's why, when we recite certain healing prayers in English rather than Hebrew, the prayer doesn't have its full power.

Even though the Hebrew words can be translated into English, their vibrational energy forces cannot. This is why I have transliterated all the healing prayers in this text, so we can receive the healing vibrational effect of these letters by reciting them aloud. *The sound and vibration of Hebrew letters can create profound healing* — this is a great Kabbalistic healing secret.

In this text, we also offer Hebrew mantras to bring about physical healing through the vibrational forces in the pattern and order of words.

Of all the Jewish holidays, the religious holiday that best celebrates the mystery and magic of the Hebrew language is *Shavu'ot,* known also as Feast of Weeks or Feast of the Pentecost. Though *Shavu'ot* corresponds in the liturgical year to the celebration of Pentecost, it is not an equivalent to the Christian celebration. *Shavu'ot* is the holiday that commemorates God's giving of the Torah to the ancient Hebrew people. Included in the Torah reading for that day are the Ten Commandments.

These commandments correspond to the Hebrew phrase, "God said," which appears ten times in the opening pages of the Torah. These ten phrases, "God said," also parallel the ten *Sefirot.* So, inherent in the Ten Commandments that we read on *Shavu'ot* are the instruments with which God created and creates the Universe. These are the Hebrew letters and the *Sefirot,* which are the DNA of everything created.

There is a magnificent meditative spiritual exercise that is done with the first Hebrew word of the Ten Commandments — *Anochi* — which means "I." "I am the Lord your God who brings you out of the land of Egypt, out of the house of bondage" (Exodus 20:2). Reciting *Anochi* as a mantra, with special emphasis on *Ru'ach*, breath or energy, heightens vibrational cell activity, which aligns/identifies the meditator with the Presence of God.

The mantra *Anochi*, pronounced in three syllables, *ah-no-khey*, greatly energizes the human body. This is so because of the unique forces in the letters that make up the Hebrew word, and because the unique vibrations of the sound of *Anochi* have tremendous power. The articulation of this word resonates with many of the *Sefirotic* energies of the human body and leads to cellular balance and health. This first word of the Ten Commandments can be used as a mantra to be said every day before your healing prayers. This mantra has enormous healing power. More on this later.

HOW TO: How to Identify the Inner I with the Greater I

Find a comfortable place and use this room, or part of this room, as your holy sanctuary. You should meditate in the same room every day, as then you will increase the energy in that place. The ancient Kabbalists call such a special place your *mi'at meekdash — small holy place.*

1. Sit comfortably in a chair with your back upright and your feet on the floor. Loosen any belt or tie or clothing that might bind you. Close your eyes.

2. Focus on your breath. Be aware of your inhaling and your exhaling. Do this for about two minutes.

3. Breathe in gently, slowly and deeply, through your nostrils a long breath. Hold your breath for a few seconds and, as you exhale through your mouth, pronounce the *ah* sound, feeling it vibrate deeply in your belly.

4. Breathe in gently, slowly and deeply, through your nostrils a long breath. Hold your breath for a few seconds and, as you exhale through your mouth, pronounce the *no* sound, feeling it vibrate deeply in your heart area.

5. Breathe in gently, slowly and deeply, through your nostrils a long breath. Hold your breath for a few seconds and, as you exhale through your mouth, pronounce the *khey* sound, feeling it vibrate inside of your head.

6. Do this meditation ten times.

With this meditation we identify the Inner I within us with the Greater I of the Universe, that is, the *Shechina* within us with the transcendent male aspect of God, and so we become one with God. We see ourselves and we return to the recognition that we are not alone, we are not separate, but we are one with God.

Illness is a result of a faulty *weltanschauung* or worldview that accepts the individual as separate from God. Healing happens when the individual recognizes that s/he and God are not two separate beings, that God is hidden in everything. When we recognize the unity of all things in God, we have healing. This meditation is a mantra meditation that recognizes and affirms our oneness with God.

NOTES

1. Jews are obligated to recite the *Sh'ma* prayer every morning, every evening, and at bed time. The *Sh'ma* prayer — *Hear O Israel, the Lord our God, the Lord is One* — teaches us that not only is there one God throughout the universe, but we are all One in God. We are all connected to each other.

2. The *Sefirot* are Ten Divine Creations which emanate from God to guide the Universe. Though there is a logical order to them — with *Keter* being the first of the *Sefirot* and *Malchut* the tenth and last — there is no temporal order. And actually, all the *Sefirot* come together in *Malchut*, which is identified with the *Shechina*, the Feminine Presence of God. The ten *Sefirot* are: *Keter, Chochma, Bina, Chesed, Gevurah, Tiferet, Netzach, Hod, Yesod, Malchut*. There also is a hidden *Sefira*-like energy called *Da'at*. We will elaborate on the *Sefirot* in Chapter 8.

3. *Tikkunei Zohar* is comprised of additions to the *Zohar*, written after the *Zohar* was written.

4. *Zohar*, volume II, Harry Sperling and Morris Simon, trans. (London: Soncino Press, 1970), p. 111.

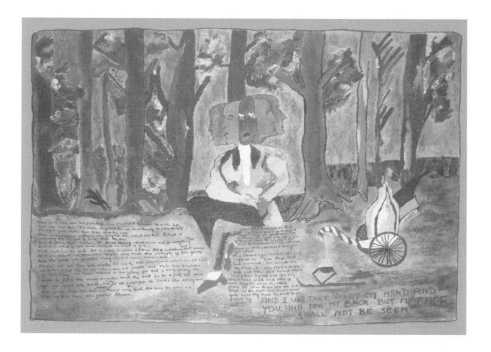

1

We Are All One

I RECEIVED a telephone call recently from a member of my synagogue whose young son had been diagnosed with a brain tumor. She was beside herself: "I know it's your vacation, Rabbi, but please, can we meet once, just once, to do healing prayer before you go back to your synagogue work?" Before I could respond, she continued, "But who am I fooling anyway? How can I pray to God? How can a good God allow my son to die? I just know he's going to die. The doctor said he's going to need surgery, and then who knows what will happen? If God is God, how could God ever allow Jason to have such a horrible thing happen to him? He's so young."

In this chapter, I will introduce you to the first prayer she and I did together, and how you can invoke it for healing body and soul in your own life. Let's begin with some background about how we have come to need and to have this prayer, its place in our tradition, and its special timeliness.

I see people every day with different types of cancer and other diseases — physical, spiritual, and emotional. I understand the power of the question that cries out from the soul: "If God is God, how can He stand by and allow my son's brain to be riddled with tumors? My son is not even twenty years old."

How could there be disease if God is God? How could we suffer so many illnesses if God is God? Why do so many people come and pray with me regularly for healing, if God is God? If God is God and can do anything and everything, including creating the Universe, how did illness sneak through the back door of God's Creation?

Kabbalah teaches us that illness entered God's universe when Adam and Eve ate from the forbidden tree, the Tree of the Knowledge of Good and

Evil, *Etz HaDaat Tov va Ra*. We trace the origin of all disease to Adam
and Eve's rebellion against God. Kabbalah explains, in the *Zohar* (3:83a),
that events recounted in the early chapters of Genesis transpired on an
entirely different plane of reality than what we experience as today's world.
Until Adam and Eve ate from the Tree of the Knowledge of Good and
Evil, the world was not a physical universe as we experience it. It was a
spiritual universe, and all beings were like light-forms or thought-forms.

Adam and Eve, before their sin, were light beings who "spanned from
heaven to earth" and "from one end of the world to the other" (Talmud
Hagiga 12A). Isaac Luria, the sixteenth-century master Kabbalist, and in
my opinion the greatest Kabbalist of all time, further taught that Adam
and Eve together contained the souls of all humankind — all the people
who would ever live (Luria, *Shaar HaGilguli Hakdama* 3). They had
within them every human soul that would ever exist.

The Kabbalah teaches that when Adam and Eve ate from the Tree of the
Knowledge of Good and Evil, they caused the intermingling of good and
evil, and reality transformed. It turned inside out and upside down, reorga-
nizing itself level after level until it finally collapsed into the physical world
we experience today, where the duality of birth and death is inescapable.

We all lived within the souls of Adam and Eve as they rebelled. So, in
a sense, we participated in their decision to eat from the Tree, and "their"
sin affects us also. Kabbalah teaches that all illness, whether physical or
psychiatric, has its roots in this first sin, and that it remains part of the
human condition. If we want to eliminate death and disease from human
life, we need to repair what we have done.

Eve offered Adam the fruit. He took it in an act of solidarity with her.
When they both had eaten, they saw they could collaborate.

But let's go back a bit. Kabbalah teaches that, in the beginning, Adam
and Eve were created as a single creature with male and female halves fused.
God severed them into individuals who could meet face to face for the first
time. "And God created Adam. . . . in the image of God . . . male and female
. . . and God caused a deep sleep to fall upon Adam . . . and He took
one of his ribs, and closed up the place with flesh. And the rib which God
took from Adam He made into a woman and God brought her to Adam"
(Genesis 1:27–2:22). One half of the "Adam" spoken of in this passage

became Adam the man and one half became Eve the woman. Kabbalah teaches that the "conscious" part of Adam remained with Adam, while the "unconscious" mind remained with Eve.

Eve is intriguing. Jewish homiletical literature says that if she had been created from Adam's feet, Adam would have walked all over her. She is created from his side to be his partner and to walk next to him. In Hebrew, she's called his *ezer kenegdo,* helpmate.

In the way that Peggy and I visualize the story of the eating of the fruit, the snake approaches Eve and says, "What about that tree, lady?" Eve is wary. She tells the snake that God not only said not to eat from that tree, but also "don't touch that tree or you will die." The words about touching the tree are Eve's, not God's.

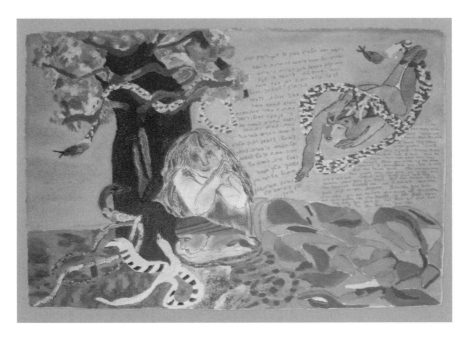

The snake says, "Lady, it's not that you will die if you eat it or touch it. God knows that when you eat of this fruit, your eyes will be opened. And you will be like gods, knowing good and evil."

Now Eve might have thought, "I don't know this God very well. I've not yet even heard God's voice myself. Why should I trust God over this snake? As a matter of fact, the snake is a good-looking fellow. That fruit looks delicious. And the tree will make me wise." Then, even though she had said, "We're not supposed to eat it *and* we're not supposed to touch it," she does both. The eye-candy fruit and the eye-candy snake who spoke so smoothly are probably what inspired her.

We imagine that Eve then untied her hair, walked toward Adam with a sexy gait, and said: "I've got an amazing piece of fruit here for you, big boy. Come try it out." And he did.

How could a snake talk? How could a snake hear and understand the voice of God? How could Adam and Eve hear the voice of God?

The Sages of the Kabbalah teach that the first human beings, Adam and Eve, spanned the distance from the heavens to the earth, from one end of the world to the other. That Adam, in which male and female were fused prior to being severed into Adam the man and Eve the woman, contained the universe. The soul of Adam was one inclusive soul. The other beings in Eden were like cells and organs within Adam's "all-encompassing body." Adam's body was made of light. Adam's soul permeated the thinking of every creature.

Hence, Adam could understand the thinking and speaking of the snake, Eve, and even the Lord God. Adam's vision encompassed and incorporated the unique contribution of every single thing. Adam's consciousness embraced the entirety of reality and united the diversity of creatures in a higher order of unity — greater than the sum of its parts.

Just as a soul pervades an entire body, Adam's soul pervaded all creation. Creation was Adam's body. Every other creature became a cell, limb, organ in this body. Every being was an individual unto itself as well as a cell in what was called *Adam HaRishon,* the first Adam. We can compare this to the cells in our own bodies, where each cell experiences itself both as a unique entity and as the person of whom it is a part.

When God asked Adam to name each creature, Adam merged with the creature as he named it. This is how Adam saw the purpose of each species, its place in the cosmic creation and its task in *tikkun*: healing, repair, rectification of the order or harmony of the universe and the individual.[1] Within the soul of *Adam HaRishon* everything was connected to everything. And of course, *Adam HaRishon* was connected with the Creator.

When Adam was first created, he was pure. His purpose was to raise the system of worlds — *Assiyah, Yetzirah,* and *Briah* — to their highest root in *Atzilut,* and ultimately into *Adam Kadmon,* which serves as a bridge to the infinite *Ayn Sof.*[2] But instead of drawing the transcendent light of the *Ayn Sof* into these worlds, Adam chose to eat of the fruit of the Tree of Knowledge of Good and Evil.

Before disobeying God, Adam and Eve lived in a world where everything was one. All the worlds were one. All the animals, Adam, Eve, God were connected. But after eating from the Tree, Adam and Eve embraced a duality of birth and death, good and evil, light and darkness, happiness and sadness. This disconnected them from the Creator, with the result that the soul of *Adam HaRishon* was disconnected from the Spiritual world and shattered into many fragments, called individual souls. The Kabbalists call this "the breaking of the soul of *Adam HaRishon.*" The soul fragmented into 600,000 root souls, which broke down into six billion individual souls.

In the Garden of Eden, Adam and Eve had "light bodies," as did all creatures; but after the Sin, their bodies and those of other creatures were clothed in material "garments of skin." No longer could Adam or Eve see from one end of the Universe to the other. This light was now hidden.

The Sin changed Reality from being a spiritual community embodied in one soul connected with God, to a reality shattered into a myriad of pieces and scattered through time and space, throughout history and the cosmos. Today our human vision does not span the distance from the heavens to the Earth, from one end of the world to the other. Creation is a broken vessel which must be repaired. Kabbalah mandates that we find each piece, brush it off, clean it, repair it, and lovingly put it back in place.

To succeed in this kind of work, we need to recover our Vision. We need to see again that the 600,000 root souls in the Universe are spiritually connected. We need to see that each of the millions of cells that comprise a root soul has its own mission and service to perform for the Creator and must come into a life all its own.

Each of us has long been a piece in a shattered puzzle that was once a single common soul. Now it is time for correction, *tikkun,* to regroup, reintegrate the pieces. This is the function of our world in this time, according to teachings of Kabbalah.

Quantum physics teaches us that the universe is not a collection of separate things moving in empty space. All matter exists in a great quantum web of connection. Nothing is completely separate. We are even connected to our enemies, as it is said that we are who we hate.

It is difficult to understand that, despite appearances, we are all connected, all really one. Though humankind's fall from Eden happened in a single bite, the repercussions of that fall were gradual and took place over thousands and thousands of years. In this devolution, each moment of the loss of consciousness of Oneness was reinforced by the moment before it.

Currently, we are in a time period called *Ikvot Meshicha,* the heels of the Messiah (Talmud B., *Sota* 49B). At this time in the spiritual history of humankind, God's Presence is so hidden that it's almost undetectable. The givers of our Torah foresaw that this time would come. And so, Torah teaches us again and again the most important tenet of Jewish faith:

שְׁמַע יִשְׂרָאֵל יהוה אֱלֹהֵינוּ יהוה אֶחָד

Sh'ma Yis'ra'el, YHVH Eloheinu, YHVH echad.

Hear O Israel, YHVH is our God, YHVH is One.

(Deuteronomy 6:4)

This declaration is called the *Sh'ma.* We say it as a prayer three times a day — once in our morning prayers, once in our evening prayers, and then again when tucked into bed just before sleep. Peggy and I recite this prayer every night, as the last thing we do together before we close our eyes. And then, each morning, we recite the *Modeh Ani* prayer (the first prayer of the day, expressing gratitude to God for the return of our souls, along with *Sh'ma.*

Reciting these prayers from our hearts revitalizes our awareness that we are all connected to each other and to God. We realize each time that even though Adam and Eve created the first step in the spiritual devolution of the world, God has never abandoned us: In the Torah that God reveals to us, we have a sacred liturgy — prayers that, when said regularly, open us to seeing that we are all connected, that we are all really one.[3]

We also say the *Sh'ma* prayer with the dying, reminding the person that he or she is not alone, but is participating with God in a new transformation. The *Sh'ma* prayer is also written inside every *mezuzah*, the small sacred containers that we Jews affix to every doorpost in our homes. This holy prayer is also in the phylacteries or *tefillin* that observant Jewish people wear on the arm and on the head six days a week while reciting morning prayers.

Through the *Sh'ma* we come to understand clearly that the single most important principle of Judaism is that God is One and that everything comes from this one source: God is the absolute One being behind everything that exists.

Kabbalah further understands this essential prayer to mean not only that God is One, but also that God is all that there is: Nothing exists but GOD.

Wow! This is the secret of Deuteronomy 6:3–5: everything that exists is part of God's absolute and indivisible unity. This Oneness precedes and transcends all existence and, at the same time, permeates all existence. This is one great Secret that Kabbalah teaches us to apply in healing. When hugging someone for healing, for instance, I hold in my mind that we are all one. The Kabbalah teaches us that even though Reality may appear to be a composite of individual units, all separate from each other, our souls are One. We are all One in God.

God is in the pencil, in our dog, in every pebble on the seashore and every stone on the mountain. God is in every human being. God is in everything and everything is in God. God is the Being that unites all of us. We are all One. There is only God.

This we affirm and remember as we fill our hearts with the *Sh'ma*.

We provide an advanced practice of the *Sh'ma* meditation in our appendix "The *Sh'ma* Meditation and the *Sefirot*," which may be useful for you when you are familiar with the rest of this book.

Healing with a Hug

There is a wonderful meditation that I often do which is very simple, based on the Oneness of all. In this meditation, I and the person I am praying with stand in front of the open Ark, recognizing that we are standing on holy ground. Holy ground does not necessarily have to be only in front of an Ark. It can be anywhere you feel God's Presence. God is wherever you let Him in. As we are hugging (see below), I remember the great Kabbalistic healing secret that we are not separate individuals; we are made up of the same stuff which is God. And, if God is within each of us from head to toe, there is no more room for illness. When our souls come together as we hug, we feel the love that we have for the person we are hugging, the love we have for ourselves, and the love we have for God. We feel that the tremendous love we have for the person we are hugging is bringing a great healing.

We recite two texts again and again, silently. The first is: *Hear O Israel, YHVH is our God, YHVH is One.* We know as we recite this that we are never alone; we are always one with the other. We are always one with God. The second text we recite repeatedly as a mantra is: *You shall love your fellow as you love yourself.* As we recite this one again and again we remember the *Midrash* or commentary to this text, which is: "You shall love your fellow because he is like yourself." We both know that I and my neighbor are made up of the stuff of God.

Gematria [4] teaches that *Ahava*, the Hebrew word for love, has the numerical equivalent of 13. And *YHVH*, the most powerful Presence of God, has the numerical equivalent of 26. We can see that:

AHAVA	+	AHAVA	=	YHVH
13	+	13	=	26

When two people hug lovingly, the Presence of God and God's light join them automatically. It's not that God says, "Now that they are hugging in love, I will reward them with My Presence." God's Presence necessarily is manifest when two people hug with love. God can't help but exist. God can't help but exist when two people embrace in love. This is spiritual physics. 13 + 13 is always 26. *Ahava* and *Ahava* is always the Presence of *YHVH*. Dan and Phyllis, a deaf couple in our synagogue, love me very much. They were with me when we began our congregation of deaf and hearing people years ago. We had fewer than fifteen families then, and I was extremely close with each of them. Dan and Phyllis had seen all their family members, cousins, uncles and aunts, nieces and nephews reach bar/bat mitzvah and get married. They had gone to various services in several synagogues, but they never could understand what was being said, because none of the rabbis used sign language in their services. When I came on the scene and conducted services in sign language, this opened their ears to Torah Judaism, and they felt a tremendous love for me, as I did for them.

Last year, Dan was diagnosed with polyps on his vocal cords. He was terrified, because even though he, like his wife, was deaf, he was trained orally. In addition to becoming fluent in American Sign Language, he had been taught to speak very well. The thought that the polyps might impair his speech was terrifying to him. He often serves as his wife's interpreter, speaking for her to doctors, insurance brokers, and others.

John, another young man, profoundly deaf, visited me after an accident in which shards of glass scratched the corneas of both his eyes. He was terrified that he might become blind as a result. For deaf persons, the possibility of blindness is even more terrifying than for a hearing person, because it would limit their communication in the world even more.

One thing that both these men had in common, in addition to their deafness, was their agnosticism. Though they loved Jewish practice and synagogue life and they loved studying Torah with me, they both often said, "If there is a God that cares about me and loves me, why was I born deaf?" This was unlike most deaf people I know, who are proud of their deafness.

These two men were terrified about how losing their speech or eyesight could make their lives even more difficult. Because of their agnosticism, however, they would not pray with me using God's energy. So I invited each of them to visit with me every week, and I would simply hug each man in front of the open Ark. As I hugged Dan, I knew that he loved me and I loved him, and I was confident that God was present. I visualized him as well and healed. And the internal dynamic was the same with John.

In one vision, I saw Dan telling me his polyps were gone. In another, I saw John telling me that his eyesight was now perfectly restored, and his scratched corneas were no more.

One thing very important to note: In our work together it was mandatory that both of them be under a physician's care, and they accepted this happily. Prayer is not meant to replace medical care. It is intended to greatly increase the efficacy of medical treatment.

If you practice healing, do your healing work in a specific place every time: That place will become holy. It will be your *mi'at meekdash,* your little sanctuary.

HOW TO: How to Pray with a Hug

1. You and the person you are praying with should sit in comfortable chairs, facing each other.

2. Visualize the room is filled with God's light. As you breathe in gently and deeply through your nostrils, imagine God's light coming into you through every pore in your body. Do this three times, and know that every organ and limb of your body is filled with God's light.

3. Both of you now stand up and hug one another. Think of your love for the person you are hugging, and his or her love for you, remembering that this automatically brings God's Presence to join you. 13 + 13 = 26. Visualize that both of you are one and made up of the same stuff we call God. As you visualize the person healthy and well, you *know* the person you are praying for is healthy and well. For example, I saw my friends with no more damaged corneas or speaking without dangerous polyps. Continue to feel the oneness, that you and your partner are one with God.

4. Repeat as a mantra, *Hear O Israel, YHVH is our God, YHVH is One,* knowing this means not only that God is One, but also *we* are all one in God. Then follow this with a second mantra: *You shall love your fellow as yourself* — recognizing that your fellow is yourself. We are all one. Repeat each mantra for a total of ten times.

5. Thank God in faith for the healing, knowing that *when you pray, you pray as if your prayer has already been answered.*

When I hug someone with whom I'm praying, I recognize and know that I am hugging God. And when I am hugging God, I feel as though I am receiving the Divine Presence, rather than only serving as an instrument delivering the Divine Presence. When I was hugging these two fellows, I felt in each case as if I was filled up with the Presence of God. If God is in me, and if I am like my fellow, then God is equally in her or him. As I hug the person, I know I am hugging God, and I feel God's Presence welling up within me in even greater amounts. Instead of giving, I am Receiving. And in Receiving, we are both doing Kabbalah and we are both experiencing healing. This is a reason why the *Amidah* prayer for healing says, *Refa'einu Adonai v'neirafeh hoshi'einu v'nivashe'ah ki t'hilateinu atah v'ha'aleh refuah shleimah l'chol makoteinu ki el melech rofeh v'ne'eman v'rachaman atah. Baruch atah Adonai rofeh cholim: Heal us, O Lord and we shall be healed. Save us and we shall be saved. Grant us a perfect healing from all our wounds. Praised is the Lord, Healer of the Sick.*

As we embrace the "other" and the "other" embraces us, we both recognize that we are one. We Receive from each other. And in Receiving, there is giving. And in giving, there is more Receiving. Somehow, the touching of our bodies activates the movement of our souls. God's spiritual energy flows into us through the person we hug or touch and through us into the person we are praying for. Because we are One.

In this prayer, then, instead of imagining that you are only delivering the Divine Presence, imagine that you are also Receiving the Divine Presence from the person you are hugging.

Say, as a mantra, two texts: *Hear O Israel, YHVH is our God, YHVH is One*, recognizing that you and your fellow are one and the same, and that wonderful prayer in the *Amidah: Heal us and we shall be healed.* You may say them in Hebrew or in English, though there is powerful energy to the Hebrew letters as we will see in Chapter 6. Saying the prayer aloud in Hebrew gives power and punch to the healing process, as the Hebrew letters are the DNA of the universe.

When I see God within the person I am praying for, I see God within myself. And when I receive the Divine Presence from that person, this heightens my sense of the Divine within myself and increases the closeness between us. This heightens our love for one another, which increases the efficacy of our healing prayer even more.

Rabbi Nachman of Breslov, the great eighteenth-century Jewish healer, teaches that the main cure for any illness depends upon *Teshuvah,* (Re-) turning. The Torah "permits the doctor to heal after turning has been made" (*Likutei Etzot,* p. 248). We need to turn toward God. We need to turn toward the recognition that we are one with the Divine. We need to turn from preoccupation with the self to an embracing of the Whole. We need to be aware that we are all connected not only to one another, but to God. We need to be aware of our own Divinity.

We need to recognize and remember that Kabbalah sees illness as arising from a faulty world view that the individual is separate from the Whole. We need to be aware that God is hidden in all things, and we need to repair the Unity of all things in God. This must be our primary outlook on the world if we want to embrace Kabbalistic healing: We need to recognize that we are holy and connected with the Divine.

There is a wonderful healing meditation with regard to all this, also written by Rabbi Nachman of Breslov. We simply say the mantra: עולם רבונו של, *Ribbono shel Olam,* which means *Master of the Universe.* My grandfathers Rabbi Sheinman and Rabbi Goldhamer preferred the Hasidic pronunciation, *Ribboini shel oylawm,* but this is an ideal healing meditation either way. It reminds the meditator that God is not only everywhere and in everything outside us, but within us completely as well.

HOW TO: *Ribbono shel Olam* Meditation

1. Pick a special room for meditation. Let this be your sacred part of the house, your *mi'at meekdash.*

2. Sit with your eyes closed and relaxed. Let your hands rest on your lap but do not clasp them together. Clear your mind of all concerns. Even sing a song if you like.

3. Repeat רבונו של עולם, *Ribbono shel Olam,* again and again, very softly. You may even whisper this mantra. But do not merely think it in the mind.

4. As you recite *Ribbono shel Olam* again and again, your internal dynamic should be that God is within you from head to toe. You are one with God completely, recognizing that the root of all illness can be traced to spiritual imbalance, mistakenly thinking that you are separate from God. Wellness depends on the recognition and the awareness that you are part of God. God is within you from head to toe. Thinking we are separate from God makes us receptive to illness. We need to shatter the ego momentarily and embrace the reality that we are One with God. We can do this by reciting Rabbi Nachman's mantra *Ribbono shel Olam.*

5. Do this for ten minutes.

Olam, the Hebrew word for Universe, is derived from the Hebrew word *alam,* to conceal. The Universe is understood as that which conceals the Divine. When a person meditates on *Ribbono shel Olam,* she is saying that "concealed or hidden within me is a Master." I like to repeat the mantra meditation *Ribbono shel Olam* mantra while looking at the *Tetragrammaton YHVH*. It is very powerful to look at the *Tetragrammaton,* or Face of God, while reciting Rabbi Nachman's mantra.

HOW TO: *Ribbono shel Olam* **Meditation with Increased Voltage**

YHVH

1. Go to your *mi'at meekdash*. Sit with your eyes closed and relaxed, hands on your lap but not clasped together. Clear your mind of all concerns. Perhaps even sing a song if you like.

2. Repeat *Ribbono shel Olam* again and again, very softly. You may even whisper it. Don't merely think it in the mind.

3. As you recite, your internal dynamic should be that God is within you from head to toe. Recall that the major root of illness is the lack of awareness that you are connected to God, filled with God.

4. As you recite *Ribbono shel Olam* again and again, visualize the Face of God, *YHVH* יֱהֵוֵה.

HOW TO: *Ribbono shel Olam* **Meditation with Increased Voltage #2**

Rabbi Yaakov shared this mystical meditative practice with me. As you recite *Ribbono shel Olam,* stare at a visual of the *YHVH* or Face of God on a piece of paper. This increases the power of the *Ribbono shel Olam* meditation.

1–3. Repeat steps 1–3 as above.

4. Now repeat *Ribbono shel Olam—Hineini, Master of the Universe, here I am,* many times. When God called Abraham, Moses, Isaiah, and other prophets, they responded by saying *hineini.* Literally it translates as "I am here." But the word *hineini* has much more meaning than its literal translation. It means "God, I am here and I am ready to do whatever You ask of me."

5. Recite *Ribbono shel Olam—Hineini* five times. Each time you say it, remember a time that God did a wonderful thing in your life. For example, when I do it I remember saving a boy from drowning

and say *Ribbono shel Olam—Hineini.* I remember my ordination in my mind's eye, and I say *Ribbono shel Olam—Hineini.* I
visualize my marriage to Peggy in our temple and look back with
thanks and say *Ribbono shel Olam—Hineini.* As I repeat *Ribbono
shel Olam—Hineini,* I recognize that God is within me today as
much as He/She was within me yesterday, and that God's Presence
yesterday and today are One.

NOTES

1. We develop the theme of *tikkun* as this book progresses.

2. The Kabbalah teaches that there are five parallel or simultaneous "worlds." These
   worlds, from "lowest" to "highest," are *Assiyah,* the physical reality which we experience;
   Yetzirah, the realm of Formation; *Briah,* the realm of Creation; *Atzilut,* the realm of
   Emanation; and *Adam Kadmon,* which is an intermediate world between the lower
   worlds and *Ayn Sof.* These are spiritual levels of creation that give us an understanding
   of the profound texture of the Universe and a greater awareness of God. They refer as
   well to states of consciousness. When we enter a different world, we embrace a different
   state of consciousness. We give more information on these worlds in Chapters 8 and
   19.

3. Kabbalistic writings teach that there was one time in world history that almost brought
   us back to Eden: when God revealed His Torah on Mount Sinai. Kabbalists see this
   revelation as the single greatest manifestation of God on Earth. It reversed the damage
   of the sin of the Tree of Knowledge and restored the community of Israel to the level
   of Adam and Eve before their sin. The corruption inherited from the serpent and the
   tree and the first sin was removed. The collective healing that the Israelites experienced
   even conquered death. "If Israel had not transgressed with the Golden Calf, the Angel
   of Death would have lost all power over her" (*Shemot Rabba* 32:1).

   The Sinaitic Revelation released the Jewish nation from mortality and all manner
   of illness. "When the Israelites left Egypt, there were many ill and injured from the
   oppressive conditions they had endured while slaves in Egypt. At Sinai, God sent angels
   to heal them of all their ills so that their disabilities were reversed: the blind saw . . .
   the deaf heard . . . the mute spoke . . . the crippled stood. God's healing light restored
   their bodies and souls to a rectified state that was like new" (*Midrash Tanchuma,* Yitro,
   8).

4. In Hebrew, every letter has a numerical equivalent. *Gematria* is the name of the
   Kabbalistic science that uses the numerical values of Hebrew words to understand and
   decipher hidden meanings in Hebrew texts.

Spiritual Laws

At almost every bar mitzvah or wedding reception I attend in my home community of Chicago, I meet new people. Many are familiar with my work and ask questions about Kabbalah and healing. Often someone I've just met says something like this: "Rabbi Goldhamer, I'm not a religious person. I don't keep kosher. I don't go to the synagogue on Shabbat. I don't study Jewish books. But I'm a very spiritual person."

When I first heard such statements many years ago, I was surprised that people would say such a thing to a rabbi. I thought it was their way of saying, "I don't need Judaism because I'm above it. I can hook in directly to God." But after a while, I realized that when people tell me they're spiritual, they're not trying to be offensive. They just feel comfortable sharing a deep-seated intuition that they embrace and nourish.

This universe in which we live and breathe is governed not only by the rules of Newtonian and subatomic physics, but also by spiritual laws that existed when God created this universe. God Himself is bound by them. Each of us is hardwired to spiritual principles that govern this universe and everything in it.

Many of us can intuit this. We may not have the vocabulary to express it, but we can intuit it with the same certainty that we know we have to breathe to live. Possibly because I'm a rabbi, some people who know this want to share their spiritual insights with me.

A question I often hear is, "Do Jewish people believe in heaven?" Or, "Do Jewish people believe in angels with the same certainty that Christians do?" If by heaven people mean angels playing harps, or fraternizing with family members and friends who have died, Judaism does not deny that, but also does not embrace it with certainty.

Judaism does embrace the idea that when you die in this world, you will be reborn in another world: when you leave this reality, you will embrace a new reality. We believe in the eternity of the soul; and that the individual soul participates in an infinite number of realities. If we want to call the transformation from one level of reality to another level of reality "going to heaven," then Judaism believes in heaven. You might not be able to visit heaven and sit down with your grandfather, but that doesn't mean there's a total disconnection between the level of reality your grandfather enjoys and the level of reality you experience. Einstein taught that energy is neither created nor destroyed, and Kabbalah teaches that everything is made of energy. So for us it is possible that you can see your grandfather or experience him again.

When someone dies and I officiate at the funeral, I encourage the immediate family to say prayers for the deceased every day for a period of eleven months, as is Jewish custom. I also encourage them to visualize the deceased, to see her or him with their mind's eye and to speak to that person every day. This interchange of love gives increased *Ru'ach,* or energy, to the deceased.

There is no disconnection between the multiple worlds that exist in this vast geography called the Universe. In fact, there are deep spiritual connections between the different levels of reality or worlds. People feel these spiritual connections. They intuit them. That's why some can say, "I'm not religious, but I'm very spiritual."

Kabbalah strongly maintains that there are different levels of reality and spiritual connections between them. This is the mystical secret expressed in what we call the *Law of Correspondence.* Succinctly stated, it means "as above, so below; as below, so above." Whatever is true on one level of reality has a corresponding truth on every other level.

In high school physics, I learned the well-known principle that every action has an equal and opposite reaction. When I studied psychology in college, I learned that there is a corresponding principle in the psychological realm: every experience leaves its mark and impression on the personality.

In rabbinical school, the rabbis repeated again and again that, in the spiritual realm, all acts of all creatures are noticed and remembered by God.

Furthermore, nothing is at rest. There is constant movement in each realm. Biology teaches that humans and animals are always moving, digesting, aging. Physics teaches that atoms and molecules are constantly moving. In the spiritual realm, there is a continuous process of vibration.

Kabbalah teaches that before creating the universe, God had a vision of its final form, its completion. Rabbi Menachem Nachum of Chernobyl, an eighteenth-century Kabbalist, wrote in his great mystical commentary on the Torah, *The Light of the Eyes,* that healing preceded the world into existence. Can you imagine that? Even before Creation, God had a vision, an image, within Him of everyone's healing.

Rabbi Nahum's Kabbalistic theory maintains that God's vision of the future of the Cosmos included not only the vision of the Universe as a whole, but also the perfection and healing of every individual being — of you and me and all the generations of peoples that would ever be. We learn that this Divine vision inspires the Creator to create continuously.

Rabbi Isaac Luria taught that there arose a desire within *Ayn Sof,* the Infinite, at its very center point, to create the Universe. Within this desire was, and is, a vision of the final perfection of the Creation. This vision inspires God's creative process even at this very moment. The single most compelling desire is God's for the perfection of creation, including the perfection of every individual. This is the secret of Divine Providence of the Individual.

This Divine Providence embraces a kind of spiritual physics. Many Eastern religions teach that "what goes around, comes around." Everything is within the system. What we do in this life governs what will happen to us in this life or the next, or to our descendants in the future. Cause and effect also reflects the Law of Correspondence. Just as there is cause and effect in the physical world, there is cause and effect in the spiritual world, which Eastern religions call karma.

Jewish people have a version of karma, called *hashgaha pratit* in Hebrew. We also believe in an almighty merciful God, and that there is one day during the year, Yom Kippur, when we can appeal to God to suspend or modify or cancel our bad karma. If we fervently promise to pray during the coming year, to live by good deeds, *mitzvot*, and be charitable, *tzedakah*, it can happen.

This process of consciously choosing how we are to live is the primary means by which God communicates with us. Every moment He gives us a chance for growth. Prayer makes this growth process possible. When we pray, we accept that God's vision is greater than ours. This allows for God's vision to be perfected and realized.

The Law of Correspondence

What you want, the healing you desire — whether it be spiritual or physical healing — is exactly what God desires for you. The healing you want for yourself is a glimpse of God's vision of your perfection. "As below, so above. As above, so below." This is the Kabbalistic secret of the Law of Correspondence.

Kabbalah teaches that your desire, your will, your prayer for healing — this voice of your inner longing — is God speaking to you. God wants us healed. God treasures healing, now and since even before He created the Universe. This mystery is at the heart of a sacred secret of Kabbalistic healing that we mentioned earlier: *When you pray, you need to pray as if the prayer has already been answered.*

God's most powerful desire is for the perfection of His creation, which includes our own perfection and healing. This is the secret of Jewish karma, *hashgaha pratit*. As we pray, do good deeds, and do *teshuvah* (explained below), we are finding our place and our purpose in God's Plan. Kabbalah teaches that we are given the Torah, the Five Books of Moses, not only as an early narrative of our history, and not only as a textbook of God's ethical laws and statutes, but as a mystical sacred text of spiritual physics. Our Torah teaches how we can nourish our soul, and what actions in our life lead to positive and enduring effects. It teaches a kind of Jewish karma, revealing the science of cause and effect as it applies to the world of Spirit, including the Kabbalistic secret of *hashgaha pratit*. *Hashgaha pratit* reveals not only God's Presence in our lives, but also a corollary to the Law of Correspondence.

God Is Our Mirror

Another Kabbalistic secret is that God's Presence in our lives is like a mirror. How God acts toward you mirrors how you behave toward others. God will only respond to you in the same way that you respond to others.

When I teach about Kabbalah's relationship to spiritual and physical healing, I say again and again that if we want God to respond to our prayers for healing, or for anything for that matter, we need to act in a Godlike manner in this world. We need to be extra generous to the poor who ask us for money. We need to be extra kind to those who ask us for help. We truly need to be good if we want God to be good in our lives because, as the great Baal Shem Tov, one of the great mystical healers of early modern times, taught — God is our mirror.

God will reflect back to us only what we do in this world. That's the function of a mirror, to reflect. God reflects us to ourselves for our benefit. God is looking back at you when you look in this mirror, so be the kindest person you can be.

You may say, while reading this book, "There's so much to learn to become a healer. There are so many techniques and modalities that I have to acquire and practice and study. How can I do this?" You can: Just look in the mirror and understand that is where God resides, not on some mountain in the sixth level of heaven, not in the cathedrals and great synagogues of Europe and America. God lives in you.

If you want your prayers and healing blessings and mystical meditations to be efficacious, look in this mirror and bring God out of yourself into the hustle and bustle of this world. This can only happen if you are kind, because that's exactly what the *Shechina* or the Inner Presence of God is. She is Love, simple and pure love.

God Needs Our Blessings

For our healing prayers to be efficacious, we must focus on how the *Shechina* suffers with all those who suffer. This because when we pray for the *Shechina,* we become a vessel drawing in Divine Light. We also need to elevate the *Shechina* in our prayers. We need to liberate Her from Her exile and do *teshuvah*, restoring Her to Her rightful place within the

Godhead. We need to pray for God if we want healing from God. We need to bless God again and again.

A remarkable story in the Talmud (*Berachot* p. 7a) reveals the depths of God's compassion and love, and teaches that we need to bless God again and again. Reb Ishmael ben Elisha speaks:

> "It happened that I entered into the innermost part of the Sanctuary of the Holy Temple to offer incense, and I saw Akathriel, the Lord of Hosts, who was seated on a very high throne. The Lord said to me, 'Ishmael, my son, bless me.'
>
> "I answered, 'May it be Your will that Your mercy suppress Your anger, that Your mercy overcome all Your other attributes, so that You may deal with Your children according to the attribute of Mercy, and that for their sake, You stop short of the full measure of strict justice.'
>
> "And God nodded His head to me."

This text is amazing. The great Rabbi Ishmael, the High Priest, enters the innermost part of the Sanctuary, which only the High Priest can enter. Jewish theology teaches that this space, the Holy of Holies in the ancient temple, is where the Divine Presence has been most fully intuited. The High Priest can only enter it one day of the year, on Yom Kippur, the holiest of days.

The High Priest first prepares for entering this space by praying and meditating. Inside, he makes the incense offering with incense that has an extraordinarily powerful fragrance. In this Holy of Holies the High Priest becomes completely aware of the Divine Presence.

When the Divine Being, in the Talmud story, asks Rabbi Ishmael to bless Him, He does not mean that Rabbi Ishmael should utter praises on His behalf. As Rabbi Chaim of Volozhin, the great Kabbalist of nineteenth-century Vilna, explains in his major work, *Nefesh HaChayim,* blessing does not mean praise. The purpose of reciting a blessing is to increase our awareness of God in Creation. Blessing is a kind of prayer, a request. A blessing draws *potentiality* into *actuality*.

Rabbi Chaim of Volozhin further teaches that when one blesses, one touches the inner truth and purpose of another person and brings it out into this world. A blessing speaks to a person's hidden purpose. When someone blesses another, he or she activates that purpose so that it might become a reality in this world. Blessings are powerful. When one person blesses another, it's as if the person blessing reads the other's soul purpose and prays for it to be realized in this world. When you bless another, you pray that the person's precious hidden secret and sacred agenda will be realized.

When Rabbi Ishmael blesses God, he looks into God's soul and blesses, "May it be Your will that Your mercy suppress Your anger, that Your mercy overcome all Your other attributes, so that You may deal with Your children according to the attribute of Mercy, and that for their sake, You stop short of the full measure of strict justice."

And God nodded His head to Ishmael.

How did Rabbi Ishmael understand and have the insight that this should be exactly God's blessing? Rabbi Ishmael must have been on the mark, because God gave him His approval when He nodded His head. Rabbi Ishmael, among the Talmud's greatest scholars and religious leaders, understood that the deepest truth in God's soul was God's desire to do good for us.

Remember, a blessing is what happens when someone looks into the depths of another's soul, sees that person's potential, and then speaks this potential into actuality. Rabbi Ishmael saw that God's soul cries out to do good. This is the potential in God's soul, to do good and be merciful. Rabbi Ishmael knew that God's soul needed a blessing to be actualized. He knew that prayer is not an attempt to overpower God and force Him to do our will. And so it is that when we pray for another, we are really blessing the other, asking God to grant in actuality what exists in potentiality for that person.

Healing Already Exists in Potential for Everyone

Recall the teaching of Rabbi Menachem Nachum of Chernobyl that all healing of all illnesses, for all people, preceded the world into existence. In his commentary on *Chaye Sarah* he writes, "God creates the healing before the illness. Healing already exists in potential for everyone." Rabbi Menachem maintains that it is up to the person who blesses the injured or sick person to bring this healing from potentiality into actuality.

A person who truly blesses with faith understands this. When we bless another who is ill, we see wellness in that person's soul and bring that wellness into actuality through healing prayer. Remember this great Kabbalistic secret that *all healing preceded the world into existence.* Healing is already there, waiting for a blessing of faith to draw it out.

Rabbi Ishmael understood the Kabbalistic teaching that God is our mirror. Because he saw that love is what inspires God to create the universe, he also saw that the prayer of God's deepest soul is to bestow loving kindness on His creatures. Mysteriously, God needed Rabbi Ishmael's blessing to bring into actuality the love and compassion and mercy that already existed in the Soul of Divinity.

The secrets of Kabbalah are really insights into how the universe works. Kabbalah is a huge textbook of spiritual physics that explains the underlying science of spiritual law. It teaches us how to achieve and exercise soul muscle, and how to stay away from that which harms. Besides revealing spiritual cause and effect, the rules of the Spiritual Universe, it also can be understood as a deep study of the mind of God — how to establish an ongoing relationship and friendship with God, and influence the mind of God.

Blessing and Balance

Rabbi Chaim, in *Nefesh HaChayim,* maintains that to bestow blessings upon men and women is inherent in God's nature. He says that God has a basic desire to cause divine abundance to envelop us. He also says that God Himself is bound by the spiritual laws that He has brought into being, just as we are. For that reason, even though God desires that Divine abundance should fall upon the world, this can only happen if people create a world that is deserving of such blessing, with everything in harmonious balance.

The principle of *Tiferet* or Balance inheres in the Spiritual Laws that govern the Universe. We receive Divine Blessings only if we deserve them. We cannot simply reach out and create for ourselves a blessed life if this is not our due. This spiritual principle of balance comes about through the power of the *Sefirot,* out of which a world develops and comes into existence.

In the diagram of the *Sefirot* known as the *Etz Chayim,* or the Tree of Life, there is a left column and a right column, mediated by a middle column in which *Tiferet,* Balance, has a central position. *Tiferet* is the spiritual principle that inspires the creation of a world that is deserving of God's blessings of Divine Abundance.

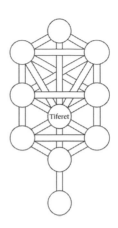

Let me be more concrete with an example of how we may create ourselves into a person deserving of Divine Abundance, or not. We learn in Talmud *Berachot* 35b that if a person enjoys a meal without saying a blessing, it is as if this person stole from God. In other words, a person who does not say a blessing before a meal does not deserve the meal. Rashi, who lived in eleventh-century France and was one of the greatest Jewish interpreters of the Talmud and Bible, explains that "stolen from God, means God's blessing was stolen." One would think that it is the *meal* that is stolen by not saying the blessing. Nonetheless, Rashi says that God's "blessing" is actually what is stolen.

There is a teaching which says that God created the physical universe to enter into a relationship with human beings. In the beginning, there arose a "desire" within the *Ayn Sof,* or God, to be called by His names. But how could God be called The Compassionate One or The Merciful One or The Great One, for example, if there were no one to whom He could show compassion or mercy or greatness? Because the desire to express goodness, mercy, and love is what inspires God to create the physical universe, God must bring into actuality people who can benefit from goodness and mercy and love. When people call God by Divine names and develop a close relationship with their Divine Source, Divine Abundance flows. This is hardwired into the universe from the beginning.

In contrast, if people leave God, refrain from calling God by His names, refrain from praying to and talking with God, and so become distanced from God, Divine Abundance ceases to flow abundantly. God wants Abundance to flow, but it can only flow if people maintain an ongoing relationship with Him. This spiritual principle is just as real as the physical principle of gravity.

Let's combine this understanding with what Rashi teaches about a person who eats without saying a blessing. He says that such a person has "stolen God's blessing, because this person has stolen the ability for God to rain His blessings upon us." Remember that a blessing is what activates sacred potential in another and brings it to actuality. So when we fail to say a blessing to God before eating, we fail to activate the potential of the Divine Desire to rain abundance upon ourselves and the world. God's potential does not become actualized. We deny God the opportunity to rain divine blessing upon us: we steal from God.

A blessing is like a key; when you turn the key, the door opens. This is a spiritual principle that governs the universe. We deny God from actualizing the flow of Divine Abundance when we don't offer blessings appropriate to an occasion. We steal from God that which is most precious to Him, His ability to shower us with His love and abundance. Kabbalah calls out this point again and again: If we want to participate in the Divine Abundance stored up for us, we need to give blessings again and again. If we want to Receive Divine Abundance, we need to Give. There needs to be balance.

Prayer is not a mumbo jumbo of words that make us feel good or, at best, make us aware of the situation in which we are placed. Prayer is a powerful instrument that God has given us to unlock treasures in the spiritual worlds that have been hidden inside us for thousands of years. When you use the spiritual key of faithful prayer — to pray as if your prayer has already been answered, and it has, because the healing of all diseases was created before any of its correlate diseases appeared on Earth — you unlock the locked-up healing. What a secret! What a gift! What a loving God!

When I was growing up in Montreal, I had a wealthy aunt, Celia. She was very kind to our family, always showering us with gifts for every holiday. My mother Jean pushed us either to call Aunt Celia or to write her thank-you notes each time we received a gift. I remember saying to my mother, "But I'm only ten. How can she expect a letter from me?" But my mother insisted, "First, it's important to show gratitude for what she gave you. Second, if you send Aunt Celia a thank-you note, she will continue to send you gifts." My mother was right. It's human nature. We are hardwired to respond kindly to those who praise us and love us. As we are made in the image of God, so is God hardwired to respond in kind. When we bless Him, He will bless us back. "As below, so above. As above, so below."

Every time I eat a meal, or even a roll, I say the blessing, *Baruch atah Adonai eloheinu melech ha Olam, ha-motzi lechem min ha'aretz, Praised are You, O Lord our God, King of the Universe, who brings forth bread from the Earth.* This is a traditional Jewish blessing. Any blessing you say from any tradition (or no tradition) that stems directly from your heart is equally embraced by God, if you say it with *kavvanah.*

We humans and God are parts of a single organism. How much blessing comes from above depends on how we relate to God here on Earth. We are the jewel in the crown of God's creation. He has invested us with enormous power.

The Miniature Universe

Another Kabbalistic secret we need to know before learning these meditations and prayers for healing is that *the human body is an exact miniature replica of the entire universe.* The great Hebrew scholar Malbim writes that in the same way as the human body contains numerous openings, channels, passageways, arteries, and veins, Creation may likewise be seen as a system of channels, pipelines, and vessels though which the Divine Abundance flows to all the worlds. Creation is called *HaAdam Hagadol,* the Great Man. And Man is called *Ha'Olam Hakatan,* the Miniature Universe. This correspondence between the Universe as a whole and the human body in particular is another profound secret of how God interacts with human beings through the Spiritual Universes to bring healing to specific persons.

The human body is the temple of the soul, and corresponds to God's Light within us. As Solomon wrote in the Book of Proverbs: *Ner Adonai Nishmat Adam,* "The Light of the Lord is my soul" (Proverbs 20:27).

Divine Abundance and blessing flow through a system of channels to each one of us, depending on our actions. The more compassionate we are, the more generously we act, the more kindness we show, the more light and more blessings flow down from above. If we are worthy, our meditations and our heartfelt prayers rise up and are embraced by God, and blessings in abundance reach us. This is the power of blessing. But if we are not worthy, if we don't share our love and give on a regular basis, Divine blessings will be restricted. God's Presence will become much more hidden in our life.

The body's various systems are in constant motion, running and returning. Blood flows out of and into the heart, to and fro through every part of the body. Life-force pulses throughout the body. Everything is in motion, except when there is a blockage and different organs aren't working well. Blockage may also occur between the soul and the body. When we offer heartfelt prayers and sincere blessings regularly and act with love and compassion toward other people, this opens up the blockages between soul and body, and allows us to receive God's blessings from on high.

Here is a wonderful meditation that opens the individual soul to be identified with the soul of God. When the microcosm and the macrocosm are in sync and joined together as identical, spiritual blockages are opened.

I often do this meditation before I go to the synagogue. It reinforces my conviction that God and I are One. By welcoming the Presence of God within me, I am able to share God's Presence with my congregation in healing prayer. This spiritual meditation is a wonderful healing practice.

HOW TO: Rabbi Dan Dresher's Candle Meditation

1. Find a comfortable and restful place where you will not be disturbed, your *mi'at meekdash,* if possible, and make yourself comfortable. Loosen any tight-fitting clothing.

2. Put a candle in a candle holder, light it, and face the candle. Sit about four feet away from it. Recognize that the candle represents the light of God.

3. To practice the Presence of God, you will eliminate the "space" between you and the candle. You want to be one with God. So, with your eyes closed, visualize the candle coming closer and closer to you.

4. As you do this visualization, recite as a mantra Proverbs 20:27: *The Light of the Lord is my Soul.* If you would like to say the mantra in Hebrew, the Hebrew words are *Ner Adonai Nishmat Adam.* Say this mantra again and again with *kavvanah,* until the light of candle, the Light of God, is within you, in the middle of your torso or *Tiferet* area.

5. When you and the Light of God are one, the microcosm and the macrocosm are one. You have eliminated the separation between you and God. You are filled with the light of God.

6. Intuit this feeling of being filled with God's light. Know that you are filled with God's light. Repeat several more times, *The Light of the Lord is my Soul.*

One morning, Rabbi Yaakov Dresher took me to a baseball game that his son was playing in. I was surprised, I never expected this Hasidic rabbi to take me to a ball game, nor to discuss baseball with me. When I said this to him, he laughed. He told me that God is as much on the baseball diamond as He is in the synagogue. He quoted the great Kotzker Reb, Rabbi Menachem Mendel of Kotz, who taught "Where is God? Wherever you let Him in."

Rabbi Yaakov's son Chaim came to bat and hit a home run. The person next to us shouted *"Baruch HaShem!"* which means *Praised be the Name of God.* Later that day, during supper, Rabbi Yaakov reminded me that the reason we feel God when we hit a home run is because God is part of us.

Rabbi Yaakov asked me then if I remembered the candle meditation I had written of in my first book. He pointed out that it would be more hard-hitting (I was amused by his baseball imagery) if I put some *Ru'ach,* spirit into it. He said, "In your meditation, you bring the candle into you, thus eliminating the Spiritual Divide. But if you use your imagination, you will see that the flame of the candle only occupies the torso area of your body, or *Chesed, Gevurah,* and *Tiferet.* The meditation would be stronger if you could imagine your whole body, from *Keter* to *Malchut,* filled with light, from head to toe."

He said, "Once you see the candle burning within the torso area, take in some *Ru'ach,* and watch the *Ru'ach HaKodesh,* God's Holy Light, expand. Breathe in and out several times, and you will see the *Ru'ach HaKodesh* expand so that you will be filled with God's light from head to toe."

Here is the revised Candle Meditation that Rabbi Yaakov taught me.

HOW TO: Rabbi Dr. Yaakov Dresher's Candle Meditation

1–4. As above, for Rabbi Dan Dresher's Candle Meditation.

5. Visualizing your *Tiferet* area filled with God's light, recite in English *The Light of the Lord is my Soul* or in Hebrew: *Ner Adonai Nishmat Adam.* As you recite the mantra several times, breathe in gently and slowly through your nostrils, imagining the light of the candle expanding — as you breathe in, the light expands — from *Tiferet* to the *Chesed, Gevurah,* and *Yesod* areas of your body.

6. As you exhale gently and slowly through your nostrils, see your *Tiferet, Chesed, Gevurah,* and *Yesod* areas filled with light.

7. Recite the mantra several more times as you visualize *Tiferet, Chesed, Gevurah,* and *Yesod* filled with God's light. Then, continue to repeat the mantra as you breathe in slowly and gently through your nostrils and watch the light expand upward into the *Keter, Bina, Chochma* areas . . . and down to the *Netzach, Hod,* and *Malchut* areas of your body.

8. Intuit this feeling of being filled with God's light from head to toe. Know that you are filled with God's light.

3

Modeh Ani

ONE night when Peggy and I were at home watching TV, the phone rang. Peggy answered. I could hear immediately in her voice that something was wrong: "What do you mean, he's dead? What happened? Where is he?"

It was a policeman calling on behalf of Nona, one of our dearest friends who is deaf, to let us know that her husband Rick had just passed away. We loved Rick and Nona deeply, and were devastated to hear that he was gone. Just forty-eight hours before, the four of us had shared an extraordinary meal at a fine restaurant in honor of their fortieth anniversary.

I remember teasing Rick at the restaurant about his great appetite, as all the lamb chops on his plate quickly turned into bones. One moment he was well, vibrant, and full of life. The next moment, he was gone.

Jewish tradition gives us a prayer that recognizes the transitory nature of our lives here on Earth. During the day, we are alive and vibrant, with our souls inspiring every organ of our bodies. At night, during sleep, we believe our souls are in the heavenly world with God. Upon awakening in the morning, we thank God for returning our souls to us.

We do not take awakening or life for granted. Every Jew is asked to recite upon waking from sleep a prayer called the *Modeh Ani*, which means in English "I thank." We recognize with this prayer that the gift of our soul, from the Source of all souls, is amazing and great. Upon awakening we thank the Source for this great gift by praying: *Modeh (feminine: Modah) ani l'fanecha melech chai v'kayam shehechezarta bi nishmati bechemlah rabah emunatecha.* In English it would be something like, *I thank you with my very being, living, enduring King, for restoring my Divine Soul to me in compassion. You are faithful beyond measure.*

I find this prayer very important because I do healing prayers with people every day and need to feel connected to the Source. There are other meditations that I rotate from morning to morning because they also connect me to the Source and activate my awareness of God's Presence within. But the *Modeh Ani* prayer is a constant, connecting me to the Source every day.

This mystical *Modeh Ani* prayer is a sure way to keep you and God connected every day. It's a short, but extremely powerful way of saying thank you to God for the gift of your life.

Last week, Peggy and I exchanged gifts. She bought me a Hebrew book on a Kabbalistic theme, and I gave her a beautiful bouquet of flowers. It wasn't one of our respective birthdays or our anniversary. Giving and receiving gifts just draws us even closer to one another and helps us feel even more thankful for each other. It deepens our love for one another.

If this is true with human relationships, it is also true for relationships between God and His children. When God gives us something, we are drawn closer to Him. Every morning God gives us something enormously precious.

When we go to sleep, our soul travels to the celestial worlds. When we wake up, God gives it back to us. Our soul is not only the amazing substance that allows our brain, heart, liver, kidneys, lungs, and blood flow to work, it also is that bit of eternal life that nestles in our physical bodies as we experience this Earth. Our proper response to this gift is sincere thanks and love.

When our friend Rick died, we saw again how we can't take life for granted. It is so important that we connect with our sense of gratitude every morning, that we acknowledge every morning the Source who gives us life. But acknowledgment is not enough, thankfulness is the key. We need to acknowledge and thank our Source before we begin each day.

The prayer begins with three words, *Modeh Ani L'fanecha.* In Hebrew *Modeh L'fanecha* means "I thank you." The pronoun "I" is included in the verb, so *Modeh* is translated "I thank." The Hebrew word *Ani,* though translated "I," in this context can be translated as "the essence of my being." Therefore, I would translate *Modeh Ani L'fanecha* as "I thank You with my *Ani,* with the Essence of my being." The mystical theology of this prayer teaches that my *Ani* is my self, to the extent that my self derives from God's Self, God's *Ani*. Literally, the word *Ani* means "I."

Theologically, there is the small "I" within us, and there is the large or great "I" generally considered outside of, or beyond us. The great I is the God Transcendent. The small I is the God Immanent. So, when I recite this prayer, I recognize that my *Ani* is part of God. I am part of God, a physical part of the Transcendent God. I am the small *Ani*. Calling God "you," I think, "You are the great *Ani*. My *Ani* is derived from your *Ani*. My *Ani* mirrors your *Ani*. And as I awake, I thank you with my *Ani*. And I thank you with my *Ani* for restoring my Divine Soul to me."

The *Ani* is our inner awareness of self, which corresponds to the lowest level of Soul, called *Nefesh*. As we explain in Chapter 8, there are different levels of Soul awareness. *Nefesh* is the lowest level, in which we are completely focused on self. A higher level of Soul awareness emerges when our soul reaches the spiritual stage of *Neshamah*, in which we are aware of our direct connection with God. *Neshamah* is a channel that connects us with God extending from above down to us. Like a spiritual umbilical cord, it transcends our physical world, reaches through the spiritual worlds, and connects to God. The *Neshamah* soul is the channel for the downward flow of the ten *Sefirot*, which become individuated as ten qualities of personality.

We are given this human life to draw down as much *Neshamah* consciousness as we can into the lives we live here. It is a great Kabbalistic secret that the more *Neshamah* consciousness we draw down from God through our spiritual umbilical cord, the stronger our soul becomes. A strong soul allows us to share spirituality or healing with others.

The *Nefesh* is our self or the I within us that recognizes God from the bottom up. *Neshamah* is that aspect of Soul that is a channel that connects us with God from God down; it is our direct connection with God. If we keep these spiritual channels unblocked and clear, our prayers will be strong and our healthy bodies will reflect the strength of our prayers.

The relationship between *Neshamah* and *Nefesh* (or *Ani*) corresponds to the relationship of light to a vessel. Kabbalah teaches that if the vessel is to attain perfection, it must receive Divine Light, which flows into it. The light of God must enter the vessel gradually, with more and more light.

The divine Kabbalist Isaac Luria teaches that the soul/light must not enter the body/vessel completely at the beginning. Only some of the soul/ light shines in the body/vessel, while the rest of the light hovers over it. Our task as humans is to refine our vessels with the little bit of light that we are given so that we can receive more and more light.

It is up to us to draw into our lives as much soul consciousness or light as we can. We do this through regular prayer, meditation, and good deeds. We need to establish a solid relationship between our *Ani/Nefesh* and our *Neshamah*. This leads to excellent health. This is a profound Kabbalistic secret of healing.

We already are aware that when we eat the right foods, sleep the right number of hours, and do the right amount and kinds of exercise, we increase the health of our bodies. We also need to be aware that soul and body are one, and that ministering to the body for good health entails ministering to the soul. We need to forge a relationship of gratitude and thanksgiving between *Ani/Nefesh* and *Neshamah*.

Neshamah and *Ani/Nefesh* are unique in each one of us. While all souls are connected with one another and with the One Source, each one of us also has a unique essence, a unique *Neshamah*, a unique *Ani/Nefesh*. When we wake each morning, our first prayer is one that thanks the Source for giving us our unique *Neshamah* and unique *Ani/Nefesh,* which renew our connection to Him. We conclude our prayer thanking God for His great faith in us — faith so great that it restores our unique soul and allows the uniqueness of our *Ani/Nefesh* and *Neshamah* to shine ever more brightly.

This is what Proverbs 20:27 means when it teaches *Ner Adonai Nishmat Adam, Man's Soul is God's candle.* We can translate this idiomatically as *The Light of the Lord is my Soul.* When we do the *Modeh Ani* mystic prayer with the recognition that God's light shines constantly in our soul through *Nefesh* and *Neshamah*, through prayer and good deeds, we strengthen the relationship between body and soul that keeps us healthy. We can give extra voltage to our *Modeh Ani* prayer by combining it with the mystic meditation of *Ner Adonai Nishmat Adam* that we learned in the last chapter.

Remember: *Neshamah* is our channel with God from the top down, and *Nefesh* is our channel with God from the bottom up. It is with our *Ani/Nefesh* that we recognize God every morning. We want to keep both channels clear and strong. We want our prayers to fly to the Source, and we want His blessings to be released and flow down to each one of us. We want God's transcendent light to flow down into that little bit of transcendence that pulses and vibrates within our finite bodies, so that the finite will be embraced by the Infinite.

We go to the gym so our bodies will be healthy and strong. We want blood to flow into and out of the heart, and to and from every part of the body. We yearn for the life force that pulsates throughout our bodies. We want all our systems to be clear and open so that we may process good nourishment from the foods we eat. We want each organ to absorb what it needs and reject what is harmful to it. We don't want blockages. We recognize the interdependence of soul and body.

Just as there are physical blockages that cause disease in the body, so there are spiritual blockages that cause disease. When spiritual blockages are opened, there can be physical healing. When *Nefesh* and *Neshamah* are working optimally, there is health.

By beginning our day with this mystic *Modeh Ani* prayer, we prevent spiritual blockage and allow spiritual flow. The free-flowing light of God gives us an amazingly energized flow of life force.

HOW TO: The Mystic Prayer of *Modeh Ani*

1. As soon as you wake up in the morning, before you put your feet on the floor and your mouth to mouthwash, recite the *Modeh Ani* mystic prayer: *Modeh (feminine: Modah) ani l'fanecha melech chai v'kayam shehechezarta bi nishmati bechemlah rabah emunatecha.* In English you would say: *I thank you with my very being, living, enduring King, for restoring my Divine Soul to me in compassion. You are faithful beyond measure.*

2. As you recite the prayer, there should be an internal dynamic, recognizing that it is with *Nefesh* or *Ani* that you welcome *Neshamah* from God. In other words, recognize that the small I within you is receiving *Neshamah* energy from the transcendent I outside of or beyond itself.

3. When you finish reciting the prayer, understand that you have opened the channels to allow a balanced relationship of *Nefesh* and *Neshamah.*

4. As you feel your whole body filling up with the Light of God, know that the Light of God completely fills your soul from head to toe, to the extent that the Light of God and your soul are one. Your inner dynamic should be such that your *Ani/Nefesh* and your *Neshamah* are in perfect relationship, that the Divine Flow of God's Life Force and Light fills your body, permeating every cell.

Most mornings, Peggy and I do the mystical *Modeh Ani* prayer together in our bed. We do the *Ner Adonai* mystical meditation later on in the morning, after our morning prayers. However, sometimes we do the mystical meditative prayer *Ner Adonai* together with *Modeh Ani* as we lay in bed. The combination is quite powerful.

HOW TO: Mystical *Modeh Ani* with Increased Voltage

1–3. Same as above, for *Modeh Ani.*

4. Visualize (do not actually light) a candle coming toward you as you say as a mantra out loud or in a soft whisper, *Ner Adonai Nishmat Adam, The light of the Lord is my soul.*

5. Visualize the candle's light entering you and filling your whole *Tiferet* or chest area.

6. Repeat the mantra and visualize your chest area filled with the light of the candle. Breathe in, gently and deeply, through your nostrils, and as you breathe in, see the light expand within you to include not only *Tiferet*, but also the areas of *Chesed, Gevurah,* and *Yesod.* (see pages 60 and 121)

7. Breathe out gently and deeply through your nostrils.

8. Do this three more times, until you are filled from head to toe with the Light of God.

9. You now are also filled with the energies of *Bina, Chochma, Keter, Netzach, Hod,* and *Malchut,* to the extent that the light of God and your soul are one. Your inner dynamic should be that your *Nefesh* and *Neshamah* are in perfect relationship and in balance; that the Divine Flow of God's Light fills your soul and permeates every cell of your body.

4

The Greater Mind

I recently met my close friend Philip for brunch. Until a few months ago, he worked as the head buyer of men's clothing for a large retail chain. When he was let go, I was very disappointed. "Where am I going to get great sweaters at wholesale prices?" I thought. I confess that I'm a sucker for sweaters, so much so that winter is my favorite season. I wear sweaters even in the summer. "The seasons do not rule me," I say.

Philip is outgoing, tall, good-looking, and a few years younger than me. But you wouldn't know it by looking at us. I've been blessed with a full head of hair and a youthful spirit. I love to ask people in restaurants and stores, "How old do you think I am?" In my fifties I used to hear "thirty-five, maybe forty." Now, at sixty-nine, I'm happy when I hear I don't look a day over fifty-five.

At brunch, Philip told me that he's very discouraged. In the three months since he was "downsized" from his company, he's had no job offers. I've introduced him to several friends, but so far no bites.

As we were enjoying our French toast, he wondered aloud why his job search has not been going as well as he anticipated. "I pray every day. I even meditate on your favorite text from the Book of Proverbs: 'Trust in the Lord with all your heart. Do not depend on your own understanding. Acknowledge Him in all your ways, then He will direct your paths'" (Proverbs 3:5). He then said, "I need to tell you that if I don't find a position soon, my family and I will have to sell our home."

I explained that he was praying the wrong way — that we must pray the way the Baal Shem Tov taught. When we pray, we are to pray *as if* our prayer has already been answered. Philip was praying with the *hope* that his prayer would be answered. But he also was praying with the thought that there was a real possibility that his prayer would *not* be answered.

I said, "You are not praying with the Greater Mind."

He asked, "What's the Greater Mind?"

I replied, "I thought you read *This Is for Everyone.*" In my earlier book on healing prayer, I quoted a passage from Rabbi Levi Yitzhak of Berdichev's *Kedushat Levi,* an eighteenth-century commentary on the Torah:

> Everyone who serves God with the Greater Mind, *Mohin de Gadlut* has no fear or trepidation of any events that may happen to him. Even though he may appear to be in trouble, he has no fear in his mind and in his heart that any harm will befall him. However, he who serves God with the Lesser Mind, *Mohin de Katnut,* fears all the events that happen to him, in his mind and in his heart, he feels fear. Because of this, external forces overpower him, and he is under their domain.[1]

Those who serve God with the Greater Mind are not afraid of difficult situations they might encounter, such as illness or financial loss. When we are in the Greater Mind, we are indifferent to external circumstances that might happen, or that even *are* happening. We put our complete trust in God.

I shared this with Philip and further maintained that we not only must pray with the Greater Mind but also with the faith of the Baal Shem Tov: Pray as if your prayer has already been answered. In this way, our prayers *will* be answered. This has been my experience. It really, really works.

A few years ago, a couple in our synagogue, Mark and Barbara, wanted to have a second child. They approached me to pray with them — not because they *hoped* that prayer would work, but because they *knew* that prayer would work. They knew people who had prayed with me, and who had taken many of my classes. They had seen the success of prayer in others' lives. They had faith that if I shared Kabbalistic prayer with them, Barbara would give birth. They truly had the faith of the Greater Mind. They wanted me to teach them the "how to."

When Barbara first called me, it was in May, several weeks before my vacation. I always take the month of July off to write, paint, and rejuvenate. "Let's begin praying in August," I said.

"No," she replied. She wanted to begin to pray with me *now,* because she had conceived her first child in June. She knew, without a shadow of a doubt, that if she prayed now, she would conceive again. She prayed with the faith of the Greater Mind as Rabbi Levi Yitzhak of Berdichev instructed.

Here is their story in her own words:

My husband and I were fast approaching fifty, with one school-age child who was begging us for a brother or sister. We had tried off and on for three years to have a second child. I had a miscarriage the year before, and had also considered adoption. But after the country we chose suddenly closed their international adoptions until further notice, we went into a temporary tailspin. After three days, I asked myself: "What do I believe?" The truth is that I believed I was naturally fertile, even at age 48, and had no interest in fertility treatments, and Douglas Goldhamer was our rabbi.

I called to make an appointment with Rabbi Douglas. It was the beginning of May 2004. He was preparing to take a month off in July. I wanted to pray for a baby. He said he would like us to begin in August, upon his return, when we could work consistently. I was clearly disappointed, and he wondered why I couldn't wait until then.

Reasons: Because I had just turned 48 (not good enough). Because I wanted to (not good enough). Because I had conceived twice in early summer and believed I could again — Bingo! It was the power of my belief that convinced him.

So Rabbi Douglas agreed to begin praying with me and Mark. On May 13, I had acupuncture at noon and met Mark at the temple at 6:00 p.m. We prayed by ourselves and with Rabbi Douglas for three weeks before we discovered that we had conceived a child the day after our first appointment!

Almost every day during the pregnancy, with his hands on my abdomen, Mark said the prayer Rabbi Douglas had taught him. In February 2005, a perfect baby boy was born to 48-year-old me!

My personal program included looking for fertility signs, a nutritional cleansing program, and Chinese medicine. Some people might think the power of prayer is questionable because all the things I tried make it hard to point to prayer. But I think our story shows that we are partners with God. We did everything we could, then prayed and let go.

HOW TO: Spiritual Exercise to Reach the Greater Mind

1. Sit in a comfortable place, in a comfortable chair, with your back upright. If possible, unbuckle your belt or loosen your pants.

2. Close your eyes and recognize that the breath of the Living God is everywhere. God is as close to you as the air you breathe. God is Breath, *Ru'ach*. Do not cross your arms or legs. Inhale and exhale deeply yet gently through your nostrils, several times.

3. Repeat Proverbs 3:5 "Trust in the Lord יהוה with all your heart. Do not depend on your own understanding. Acknowledge Him in all your ways, then He will direct your paths." Say it three times out loud, with complete belief.

4. Breathe in God's *Ru'ach* gently but deeply, through your nostrils. Even as you are breathing in through your nostrils, imagine God's *Ru'ach* entering you through your head area, your torso, right arm, left arm, right leg, left leg, and feet, through all the pores of your body.

5. There is no need to count here. Just intuit God's Breath of Life filling you up.

6. As you intuit God's Breath filling you up, really *feel* the Presence of God within you, in your head, your torso, your heart, legs, etc.

7. Release God's Breath. As you exhale through your nostrils, feel every cell in your body connecting with the Divine. Feel the Presence of God in every part of your body.

8. Repeat steps 4–7 three times.

9. Repeat five times: *I am now in the Greater Mind. And I am completely filled with the Spirit of God. I am completely in God and God is completely in me. There is nothing that can harm me.*

10. Let go and let God be your Guide for the rest of the day.

———

If you embrace this text from the Book of Proverbs, and practice it, you will no longer be in the Lesser Mind. You will be in the Greater Mind, because this text from Proverbs is the Word of God. My friend Philip did not really embrace this text. Though he said the verse diligently every morning, he was filled with anxiety and fear the rest of the day. His internal dynamic was one of disbelief. He lived in the Lesser Mind.

My friends Barbara and Mark said Proverb 3:5 every day. Their internal dynamic was one of belief. They lived by the Holy Proverb all day. They let go and let God. And they lived in the Greater Mind. This means, all day they trusted in the Lord, even when fear raised its ugly head. They did not embrace the fear. They acknowledged God in all their ways by thanking God for their souls when they awoke in the morning, acknowledging God every time before they ate, and saying a prayer to God before they retired at night. They were confident that God was leading them on their path.

When a child is born, it's a miracle. When I saw their little Zach on the day of his *bris* (circumcision) — when Barbara suggested I hold him, I truly felt that I was holding a bit of God. Here I was, holding a tiny tot on the eighth day of his life on Earth — and I knew that his life was a direct result of our prayer.

The day of Zach's *bris* was beautiful. The synagogue was filled with family and friends, as we all witnessed the first moments of his new life. Peggy and I have visited the Louvre in Paris. We've seen the Western Wall in Jerusalem, climbed the stairs of St. Paul's Cathedral in London, and visited the healing chapel of St. Joseph's Oratory of Mount Royal in Montreal. But to hold this little miracle surpassed all of those monumental moments — because when I held Zach, it was as if I was holding God.

According to the Kabbalah, we become susceptible to disease when we work and live under the illusion of separation, when we see ourselves as separate from God and from one another. When we see every being as a separate individual entity, and see ourselves as not connected, we despair. And when we despair, we disrupt the harmony of mind, body, and spirit that is essential to human wellness.

"Do not despair" is the commandment that God gives us more often than any other. It is repeated in the Torah more often than any of the 613 other commandments. Torah is warning us against the division of *part* and *whole,* warning us against the *illusion* that we are *separate* from one another and from the whole. It teaches and Kabbalah preaches that when we embrace and chase after this illusion, we welcome illness into the cells of our body. I cannot repeat too often that *the illusion of our separation from God is the origin of illness.*

The more we forget that there is only God, that we are rooted in God's soul, the more we forget our divinity and the more we forget that God is in us. The more we separate ourselves from the whole, the more we fear, the more we set ourselves up for illness.

The more we remember the deep mystical truth that we are all connected with God, and that God is within each of us, the more we make ourselves accessible to wellness. When a person returns to and embraces the true understanding of unity, that person is on the Precipice of Healing. Healing begins when he or she passionately embraces the only Reality, the original Reality, the true Reality, that we are all one with God and in God.

We need to do *teshuvah*, "to return." We need to return to the deep and sacred understanding of the ancient Kabbalah: that we are all connected and that God is hidden in all things. We need to repair the broken soul of *Adam HaRishon*. We do this by embracing the world view that we are all one in God.

When the ancient Israelites were slaves in Egypt, they had no fear of obeying Moses's instruction that they sacrifice a lamb to God for the event that came to be the first Passover. They had no fear even though the Egyptians considered lambs sacred, revered the lamb with the same reverence as Hindus venerate the cow. They had no fear of Egyptian retribution. This ragtag group of slaves did not despair when Moses inspired them to sacrifice their lambs. They recognized that each one of them had a power within that could not be challenged or overcome, that within each one of them was a Greater Being, or Greater Power. They knew that if they embraced *Mohin de Gadlut*, this Greater Mind, they would prevail.

Levi Yitzhak taught that even though the ancient Israelites were in bondage in Egypt, they achieved an inner transformation that preceded their physical freedom. This inner transformation was the radical change of each individual from the Lesser Mind — *Mohin de Katnut* — to the Greater Mind. When one is in the Lesser Mind, she despairs, she fears: This won't work; that can't work. How can I do this alone? I will never succeed. Who am I that my prayers should be answered? God is in the Heavens above, and I am here below.

But when she embraces the Greater Mind, she embraces the reality that she is not alone, but is connected with God: *There is no separation between her and God.* Her faith at this time becomes enormous, and she *knows* she will be extricated from the problems that she finds herself in. In fact, she sees herself as *already* being extricated from the situation.

HOW TO: Greater Mind Meditation

1. Go to your regular place of meditation, your *mi'at meekdash.* Do this meditation every day at about the same time. This will ensure a sense of stability, constancy, and comfort. Sit in a comfortable chair or, if you wish, you may lie down.

2. Close your eyes. Do not cross your arms or legs. Take a deep breath through your nostrils and imagine the breath flowing to your brain. When you exhale, imagine the breath traveling from your brain, throughout your body, down to your toes. Do this three times.

3. Say or think the words: *I am a wonderful human being. I am unique in creation. I have a unique purpose. Even though I have a unique soul, I am connected in a single common soul made up of hundreds and hundreds of thousands of souls, connected with one another by the Golden Thread of God. God is within me. God is within me. God is within my mind. God is within my soul. I am one with God. I am in the Greater Mind.*

4. Repeat steps 2 and 3.

I remember calling Rabbi Yaakov one day. Frannie, a woman with whom I had been praying, had become very agitated, very nervous. She had first come to see me two years earlier, after her oncologist said that there was very little he could do for her any more. He had used conventional medical treatments with failing results. In addition to visiting her psychologist regularly, she had tried two different alternative practices in different parts of the country. The tumors in her abdomen were giving her great pain. Several rabbis in the Chicago area referred her to me at that point, and we began to meet almost every week to pray together in front of the Holy Ark. We also discussed the concept of the Greater Mind.

But this most recent week, she was overwhelmed with anxiety, sadness, and fear. She was very fearful of dying, because her pain was much greater than usual. We prayed again and I reminded her that it had been two years since she came to me as a last resort. "And look," I said, "you're doing great!"

But she was afraid she was dying.

So I called Rabbi Yaakov. He reminded me of Rabbi Menachem Nachum of Chernobyl's book, *The Light of the Eyes,* and directed me to read the part on *Chaye Sarah,* the section in Genesis which talks about the death of Sarah. He specifically referred me to the Hebrew commentary on the verse, Genesis 23:1, "Sarah's lifetime, the span of Sarah's life came to one hundred and twenty-seven years." Rabbi Nachum says there that "Healing preceded the world into existence. And God always creates the Healing before He inflicts the 'blow.'"

Rabbi Yaakov then asked if I understood what that means. Before I could answer, he said that Rabbi Nachum is teaching that the power of healing is present in God, even before illness occurs. Of course I knew this. This is central to my teaching. But then Rabbi Yaakov asked me to turn to Chapter 21:1 of Genesis. I said, "We're going backwards."

He reminded me, "Douglas, you know better. There's no before or after in Scripture." According to the ancient rabbis, Scripture is not divided into past, present, and future. It is the living word that is now. It all happens Now! Rabbi Yaakov further reminded me that we had studied *Kedushat Levi* two years earlier, and asked if I still had a copy of it. I told him that I did, but would have to call him back the next day, since it was at home, not in my library at the synagogue.

The following evening, Rabbi Yaakov and I studied Levi Yitzhak's commentary to Genesis 21:1, "And the Lord took note of Sarah as He had promised and the Lord did for Sarah as He had spoken." Without going into the details of the Hebrew text, Rabbi Yaakov and I saw that when God gives a promise to do some good, we need to rely on this promise absolutely. We are to have no doubt that He will deliver His promise at the appropriate time. Furthermore, God does not think in terms of past and future. The promise resides in the potential. It is delivered from potentiality into actuality through faith.

Remember what we learned in Chapter 2 from Rabbi Chaim of Volozhin's *Nefesh HaChayim:* The purpose of a blessing is to tap the inner truth and destiny of a person, and bring it into actuality. Combine this with what we learned from Rabbi Nachum in that same chapter: The healing of every illness is stored in the world to come. So you can see that if you have faith, if you are in the Greater Mind, you can pray with your friend, knowing that all healings have already been created, in the world to come. This is the future. With faith, you can bring healing from the future into the present. You need to pray with *Mohin de Gadlut,* the Greater Mind, knowing your prayer is already answered.

This is what I shared with my friend Frannie. All Frannie needed to hear was that *Hashem*[2] had the healing to her prayer in another world. All she needed to do was to know this, believe it, and pull down her healing with the lever of Greater-Mind faith. She did, and traded in her depression for renewed faith. She even said, "I just needed to know that God still cares about my healing." She continues to pray with me regularly, and she is a much happier person.

In traditional Kabbalistic language, we would say it more like this: Healing was first manifested in *Chochma* and then in *Bina,* but then had to be extended into the unfolding of the Lower *Sefirot* where the distinctions of present and future exist. The secret of Kabbalistic healing is to *retrace the unfolding of events back to its source in Bina, where all healing exists in potential.* The person of faith recognizes that healing will come into actuality when the Hidden is revealed, and when the potential is actualized. Why? Because the prayer is already answered. It was/is answered before God created the world. And it can be brought from potentiality to actuality by reaching into the future, and delivering the Promise in the present.

Past, present, and future are all ONE with Faith. God's intention before it is manifested from potentiality into actuality remains hidden. The person of faith can offer a blessing of healing and can become a conduit to receive healing for the person he or she is praying for. This is another of the many secrets of Kabbalistic healing in these sacred verses of Genesis.

NOTES

1. Levi Yitzchak, *Kedushat Levi* (Slavuta, Ukraine, 1798; reprint: Brooklyn: Rabbi Fishmann, 1977) p. 46. Also in Goldhamer and Stengel, *This Is for Everyone,* p. 25.
2. *Hashem* is the Hebrew word that many Jews use in informal communication when discussing God or *YHVH.*

Alef Power

ONE of the greatest Kabbalistic healers was the Baal Shem Tov (1700–1760). He was known in his time as the man who could become one with God and perform miraculous healings. Though his given name was Israel ben Eliezer, he was called Baal Shem Tov: the master in the ability to use the mystical names of God for miracles and healings.

One day, a greatly respected academic scholar in Poland, Rabbi Dov Baer, went to see him. Rabbi Dov Baer was a Talmud and Bible scholar, well versed in the Kabbalah. But he was unable to do healings and miracles and wanted to know why. So he traveled to the home of the Baal Shem Tov.

The two rabbis shared tea, maybe even a little schnapps, who knows? Then Rabbi Dov Baer blurted out — he couldn't hold his tongue any longer —"I've studied Kabbalah for years, since I was a *pischer*, a novice. My teacher taught me Torah and Talmud and Bible. I even teach Kabbalah to students every Tuesday and Thursday. But I can't do even one miracle. I can't do any healing. Why? Why?"

The Baal Shem Tov told Rabbi Dov Baer that once he had driven through the wilderness for eight days, and lacked bread to feed his coachman. He felt awful that he couldn't feed his trusted servant. Out of the blue, a Polish peasant happened along and gave him some bread.

The Baal Shem Tov then dismissed Rabbi Dov Baer.

Rabbi Dov Baer was confused, and returned to the inn where he was staying. He said to himself, "I will visit the Baal Shem Tov again tomorrow. Maybe I will learn why I can't do healings, even though I have studied many Kabbalistic texts."

When they met the next day, Rabbi Baal Shem Tov told him that once, a few years ago, while traveling on the road, he had no hay for his horses. But, like a miracle, a farmer came and fed the animals with much hay.

Rabbi Dov Baer said, "What are you talking about? I want to gain insights on how to heal. And you are telling me stories about your travels."

The Baal Shem Tov responded by sending him back to his hotel.

On the third day, Rabbi Dov Baer decided to try one last time. So he went back to the Baal Shem Tov's house and knocked on the door.

The Baal Shem Tov opened it and said, "You think you are well-versed in the Kabbalah?"

"Yes."

So the Baal Shem Tov took from his bookshelf an ancient text, perhaps the oldest mystical book ever written, called *Sefer Yetzirah*. He asked Rabbi Dov Baer to read and translate a passage of the Hebrew text, and offer explanations and insights. The passage dealt with the many kinds of angels, the nature of angels, and different meditations on how to inspire angels to do healing for you.

After Dov Baer read it and expounded upon its mysteries, the Baal Shem Tov said to him, "No, no, no. You have no true knowledge of Kabbalah. Let me show you."

Then the Baal Shem Tov read the exact same passage and, before the astonished eyes of Rabbi Dov Baer, the room exploded in flames — through the blaze, he heard the singing of angels. Not only did he hear them singing, he actually saw their wings — green wings, red wings, gold wings, silver wings. He saw the angel Rafael, the Angel of Healing, in his green and purple robes. He even saw the Angel of Death, with his robes and wings of black and silver. Then all his senses forsook him, and he passed out.

When he awoke, the room was as it had been when he entered it — a room filled with books and books and books. And there was the Baal Shem Tov standing opposite him. The Baal Shem Tov said, "Rabbi Dov Baer, when you read and translated and interpreted the *Sefer Yetzirah,* you read, you translated one hundred percent correctly. But you have no true knowledge, and because of this, you can't do miracles and healings. And you don't have true knowledge because there is no *Soul* in what you know."

One of the most important secrets of Kabbalistic healing is that *you first need to learn how to make contact with Soul.* This is because Soul and

Body are one. We can't study illness and health of the human body without understanding that Soul exists throughout every pore and sinew and limb and organ of the human body. To do healing, we first need to learn how to think and meditate and love with our soul. You can read many books on the Kabbalah, but you won't learn the secrets of Kabbalistic healing if you learn only with your head and not with your soul.

In the community to which I minister, there are many mixed-faith marriages. I find the differences between what various traditions offer us at the time of death very interesting. When a member of our congregation who is Catholic is dying, for example, she calls her priest — and the Jewish spouse calls me for support.

For example, the Catholic Anointing of the Sick, formerly called Last Rites, begins with the signing of the Cross with holy water. This is meant to remind the individual of the Baptismal promise to die with Christ, so as to rise to a new life with Jesus. The priest first puts his hands on the dying person's head, and then prays while anointing the person's forehead and hands. The priest will also assure the person that the community is praying for him or her. Holy Communion may be received at this time. The priest articulates quite a bit of theology, calling for belief in Jesus and the Father and the Holy Ghost.

This is very different from the Jewish last rites. When I minister to a member of my congregation who is dying, there is no assertion of belief. I ask him or her nothing about belief. I recite Hebrew prayers, but these prayers are to remind the individual of our ancient language, ancient history, and of the millions of Jews who died before and are connected to him. I, the rabbi, have no power to release his soul from his body.

The last rites in Judaism are called the *Vidui* or confession. Though they do articulate theological ideas, they are cultural in nature. They assure the dying person that he or she is connected to Jewish communities that went before, but they don't mandate a particular set of beliefs. Also, it actually is not mandatory for the rabbi to deliver the *Vidui*. This is because each Jewish person is responsible for the releasing of his or her own soul at the time of death. No minister can do that for another person. We believe that each of us has responsibility for our own soul.

The Kabbalah teaches that, in order for a person's soul to go to heaven, *that person must have soul muscle.* Their soul must be strong enough at the time of death to break through the body. And the only way the soul can gain this strength is through developing *soul muscle.*

How do we gain soul muscle? We gain soul muscle by doing good deeds, studying Torah and its teaching, and by praying regularly throughout our lives. In other words, we gain soul muscle by learning how to give and receive with our soul, with compassion, in everyday life, by learning how to hear and receive the Presence of God in our everyday prayers and meditative practice, and by learning how to receive the Presence of God through regular Torah learning.

To study Kabbalah, to practice Kabbalah, to know Kabbalah, and to learn the secrets of Kabbalistic healing, you have to find your soul, know it, and exercise it regularly — just as, if you want a nice body, a sexy body, you have to work out. You can't buy either one in a bottle.

Kabbalah, simply put, is Judaism's inner science of how to *Receive* with our soul. As we learn this by developing soul muscle, we become better Kabbalists.

In Israel, the word "Kabbalah" often appears behind the front desk in a hotel. I remember when I first visited there I thought, "Fascinating, free Kabbalah lessons at the hotel." Peggy reminded me that behind a hotel desk "Kabbalah" means "Reception." The word stems from the Hebrew root *Kibel,* to receive.

In its traditional spiritual context, the term Kabbalah implies a certain kind of Soul Wisdom of learning how to receive. The Talmud says that Moses *kibel* (received) the Torah on Mount Sinai. He gave it to Joshua. Joshua transmitted it to the Elders. The Elders transmitted it to the prophets. The prophets transmitted it to the ancient rabbis of the Great Assembly.

Moses was the greatest of all the prophets, and the greatest Kabbalist. He was the greatest Kabbalist because the more he gave, the more he was able to receive. He was the paradigm of complete and total Kabbalah, demonstrating receptivity to the prophetic experience, including the prophetic experience of healing.

When Rabbi Dov Baer approaches Rabbi Baal Shem Tov to discover the hidden secrets of healing, the Baal Shem Tov tells him stories about his coachman and some bread, and his horses and some hay. What does this mean? It certainly doesn't sound profound. What could be more ordinary than a coachman and bread, a peasant and hay? What does this have to do with Kabbalah? Why waste time with those stories? What secret lies in those stories that teach us about healing?

This is exactly what Rabbi Dov Baer is thinking. He wants a highly esoteric explanation on how to heal. He doesn't relate to ordinary life experience. By rejecting the mystery in the ordinary, by rejecting these simple events, Rabbi Dov Baer refuses to deal with the mysteries of everyday life — things not mentioned in the Talmud. His soul could not reach beyond his mind, to receive the Divine mysteries and wonders of everyday life. Finally, Rabbi Baal Shem Tov asks him to read from an old Kabbalistic book. It doesn't seem complicated. It doesn't seem hard. Rabbi Dov Baer thinks, "I can do this. I've read more difficult passages before."

When Dov Baer reads the passage, it's the sound of words signifying nothing. When Rabbi Baal Shem Tov then reads the exact same passage, a true mystical experience takes place. Rabbi Dov Baer wants to know why, and Rabbi Baal Shem Tov looks him in the eye and says, "Because you are not connecting with your soul. You don't know how to *Receive* with your soul."

When we attend services at some synagogues today, we often leave feeling uninspired. That is because many rabbis today interpret the world through their minds. The Baal Shem Tov screams and shouts and dances and says, "True knowledge goes beyond the mind. True knowledge must be received by the soul."

Kabbalah is learning how to receive the world through your soul. If you do that, your sense of reality will change drastically. So another great Kabbalistic secret is that *we need to receive the world through our souls, not through our minds.*

We will learn how to deliver healing, but first it is crucial to understand that your soul or energy centers must first be in balance. This book teaches how to be in spiritual health yourself first, and then how, in spiritual health, you can deliver spiritual and physical well-being to another. It's all about balance. So let us next speak of *Alef.*

א – Alef

The letter Alef stood outside, but did not enter. The Holy One Blessed be He said to it: "Alef, Alef, why do you not enter and come before Me like the rest of the letters?"

The Alef replied, "Master of the Universe, because I saw that all the letters left you without any advantage, then what shall I do there myself? Furthermore, You have already given to letter Bet the greatest gift of all. And it is not fit for the Supernal King that He should take back the gift which He gave to His servant, and give it to another. The Holy One Blessed be He said, "Alef, Alef, even though the world was created with Bet, you will be the first of all the letters. My unity shall be expressed only by you. Everything the people do shall begin with you. Therefore all unity shall be expressed by the letter Alef."

—Introduction to the *Book of the Zohar,* "*The Letters,*" of Rav Hamnuna Saba

When I discovered that I had Klippel-Trenaunay, I was studying at the University of Chicago for my Ph.D. I was walking with crutches, as my many operations had made walking very painful. And I heard that a wonderful Kabbalistic healer was giving a lecture on Kabbalah in someone's home on Washtenaw Street in Rogers Park.

The lecture was in the living room. The room was crowded. I entered with my crutches and tried to find a seat. As I looked for one, I saw the lecturer staring at me. It soon felt as if everyone was staring at me. My heart was pounding. I didn't know what to do. I didn't know where to sit. Then the teacher, Rabbi Daniel Dresher, beckoned me toward him. *"Kim, kim du."* He looked so old.

I approached and he offered me an apple, holding it by the stem. I thought, why is the teacher giving me an apple? Shouldn't I be giving him an apple? Nonetheless, I reached out to take it. But the people in the room shouted, "No, no." So I withdrew my hand.

The Kabbalah teacher offered me the apple again. I went to take it, and the people shouted "No!" I think one girl felt sorry for me, because I saw her cup her hands. I took it as a sign, so I did the same, putting my hands under the apple.

The teacher said, "Good. You are doing Kabbalah. Kabbalah means 'receiving.' Kabbalah is the art of learning how to receive." He already was teaching me. When someone offers you a gift, don't *take* it. Instead, make yourself a space so that you can *receive* it. Kabbalah is about receiving life as a gift. Kabbalah is about receiving with your soul, the soul of others, and the soul of God.

Rabbi Dresher loved Hebrew. I mean, he *loved* Hebrew. He believed strongly that every Hebrew letter has a soul. He saw each Hebrew letter as a unique form of energy, which God uses. He taught me that God uses these twenty-two different energetic forces in creating the Universe. He said that God did not create the Universe at one time and stop, but uses the Hebrew letters regularly in an ongoing activity of creation.

The Hebrew letters are the instruments with which God creates. Everything is composed of them. We use them in Kabbalistic healing. We will study them in detail in Chapter 6, but it is important that we study here the *Alef* א, the first letter of the Hebrew alphabet.

Rabbi Dresher had a deep fondness for the letter *Alef*. He would say to me, "I see God when I see the letter *Alef*." If you look at the *Alef*, you will see that it is composed of two *Yods* and a diagonal *Vav*. *Gematria*, an ancient system of assigning numbers to words and letters to discover significant relationships, assigns *Yod* the number 10 and *Vav* the number 6. Together, two *Yods* plus one *Vav* — 10 + 10 + 6 — adds up 26, the same number that *gematria* yields for *YHVH* and for the Hebrew word for Love, *Ahava*. This suggests a profound inner connection between *Alef* and *YHVH* and Love.

As I mentioned, Rabbi Dresher was a Hasidic rabbi, and I am not. My usual dress is corduroy trousers, tweed sport jacket, sweater vest, button-down shirt, regimental striped tie, and saddle oxfords, all in coordinating colors. With my blond hair and tortoiseshell round glasses, I appear as a colorful person.

Rabbi Dresher wore only black and white. His shirt was white, and part of his *tallis* (prayer shawl) was white. His jacket, trousers, shoes, and hat were all black. Nonetheless, he made up for this dark dress with an extremely colorful and compassionate personality. Also, his beard was the most beautiful red beard that I have ever seen.

One day it was very hot and he had taken his jacket off. I noticed that he wore a cummerbund-like belt around his waist and I asked, "Why is your belt so thick?"

He replied, "This is not a belt, it's my *gertel*. It reminds me that the human being is the channel that unites, and separates, both heaven and Earth. It also reminds me of the first letter of the Hebrew alphabet, the *Alef*, which is known for its humility and for being a pure channel through which God's energy flows."

Rabbi Dresher continued, "When God decided to create the Universe, He contemplated with which letter He would create the world. All the Hebrew letters appeared before God. Each one argued her case as to why the Lord should begin the Creation with her. Only the letter *Alef* was silent. She presented no case. The Holy One, blessed be He, said to her, 'Why do you not present an argument of your case before me? Don't you want me to begin the Universe with you?'

"The *Alef* answered, 'I know that You have decided to begin the Universe with the letter *Bet*, since the letter *Bet* represents the Hebrew word *Berachah*, blessing, and in *Berachah* — You, Lord, are blessed. And since You promised *Bet* You would begin with her, I don't want You to take back the gift you've given.'

"The Lord then said to *Alef*, 'Even though I will create the world with the letter *Bet*, only through you do I become One.'"

Rabbi Dresher taught me that the letter *Alef*, the first of the twenty-two Hebrew letters, is so loved by God that she can be used in a meditative exercise to access God. More importantly, *Alef* can be used to fill yourself up with God's energy, so that God's *Ru'ach* becomes your *Ru'ach*. In other words, by meditating on the letter *Alef*, you can identify with the *Ru'ach* of God, and be in an excellent state to convey healing. You can become a channel for God's Healing Breath.

א

Look again now at how the single letter *Alef* is composed of three letters. There are two *Yod*s, one above and one below. Between these two *Yod*s is a slanted line, a *Vav*, that *separates* but also *unites* them (א). The *Zohar* teaches that the upper *Yod* represents God and the Upper Reality, and that the lower *Yod* represents the physical world and the Lower Reality. The slanted line that unites and separates them is the connection between Man and God. Notice that the lower *Yod* is upside down in relation to the upper *Yod*. This is another expression of the Law of Correspondence, that what is above is reflected here below: God created Man in His image.

Within the slanted line of the *Alef* is a deep Kabbalistic secret of this letter. We learn to see it not only as separating *Yod* from *Yod*, but as a connecting *Vav* that unites the Higher Reality with the Lower Reality — bringing together Man and God, or the Celestial World and the Physical (earthly) World.

Alef teaches us that when we are healthy and well and whole, the Upper Reality and Lower Reality exist in balance within us. The Upper Reality is called *Nefesh Elohit,* the Divine Soul, the divine part of our soul. And the Lower *Yod,* or Lower Reality represents *Nefesh Behamit,* the animal tendency of our soul. These two seemingly antithetical forces must be harmonized if the human being is to live effectively, fulfill his or her purpose in the world, and create soul balance, or soul muscle.

After explaining all this to me in great detail, Rabbi Dresher then taught me the following meditative exercises. The purpose of these meditations is to help you become a pure channel through which God's Celestial Energies and God's Earthly Energies flow freely. When the Upper Waters and Lower Waters flow freely, they create a balance within you. You then become an instrument of God through which you can direct healing.

א

HOW TO: *Alef* **Meditation that Allows You to Achieve a State of Soul Balance So that You Can Deliver Healing to Another, or Be in a State of Great Health Yourself**

1. As with all meditative exercises, it is important to do this meditation in your sanctuary, your *mi'at meekdash.* It's also important that you do it with *kavvanah,* knowing that God is all around you and within you.

2. Sit in a comfortable upright chair. Relax, with both of your feet planted firmly on the floor.

3. With your eyes closed, breathe in through your nostrils slowly, gently, and deeply. Be conscious of your breathing.

4. Look at the letter *Alef.* See how it is made up of a vertical *Vav* and an upper *Yod* and a lower *Yod.*

5. Study it. Visualize the *Vav* in white with a purple tinge, and the two *Yod*s in white with a green tinge. The *Alef* teaches us that we have *within our soul* an Upper Reality, *Nefesh Elohit,* and a Lower Reality, *Nefesh Behamit.* Look deeply at the *Vav* and the two *Yod*s, seeing the lower *Yod* as *Nefesh Behamit* and the upper *Yod* as *Nefesh Elohit.* Repeat this in your mind.

6. Visualizing the *Alef,* focus on the Divine Energy pulsating in *Nefesh Elohit,* the Upper Reality. Close your eyes and breathe in deeply, through your nostrils, this Divine energy. Feel this Divine energy pulsating throughout your body. As you breathe out through your nostrils, imagine this life-affirming energy flowing through every organ and limb of your body.

7. Now turn your attention to the lower *Yod* and see the energy pulsating in *Nefesh Behamit,* the Lower Reality. Close your eyes and breathe in deeply through your nostrils this human energy. Feel the human energy pulsating throughout your body. As you breathe out through your nostrils, imagine that this life-affirming energy is flowing through every organ and limb of your body.

8. With your eyes closed, as you continue to breathe in and out, feel the flow of your soul energy throughout your body. Your soul energy is your human and divine energy flowing together in balance, throughout every organ and limb of your body.

9. Continue this with your eyes closed. Breathe through your nostrils in and out, feeling the flow of your soul energies traveling throughout your body.

10. With your eyes still closed, visualize the *Alef* within you in your solar plexus area. See the white with purple tinge *Vav.* See also the white with green tinge *Yod*s. Know that this divine *Alef* is the Presence of God within you, allowing you divinity and humanity, in balance, together.

11. When you feel your soul energies are in balance, this balance not only leads to healing for yourself, but also allows you to be in a position to deliver healing.

If you are doing healing prayer with someone who needs help, it is important that you yourself be in spiritual balance before you try to deliver balance to another person. You can give only what you have. If I know that I am going to be doing lots of healing meditation with many parishioners that day, I will do a meditation for balance in the morning before I leave for the synagogue, after I do my morning prayers.

When we are healthy and well, the two worlds exist in balance within us, the Upper Reality and the Lower Reality. God and Man, the Divine and human aspects exist in balance within us.

HOW TO: *Alef* Meditation #2 So That We Are a Channel through which the Energies of Divinity and Humanity Flow in Balance

1–4. As above, for the first *Alef* meditation.

5. Look closely at the letter *Alef* on your page. Then close your eyes and imagine it as much larger, until it encompasses the complete room. See it as made of two colors, purple and green, the colors of the healing angel Rafael: The diagonal *Vav* is purple, the two *Yod*s are green.

6. Hold this image in your mind of the purple and green *Alef*— huge and encompassing the whole of your *mi'at meekdash*.

7. Focus in your mind on the lower *Yod*. Receive it as our physical world. Walk into it, don't be afraid. It is filled with green energy. Receive its energy as you are in it. This is the energy of *Nefesh Behamit,* Lower Reality — our world, our universe, our physical universe, the green Earth and the seas and the sky, all the stars and the galaxies.

8. As you receive this energy, know that there are spiritual worlds that correspond to our physical world. They are the worlds of Angels and souls, the worlds of *Yetzirah* and *Briah*. Receive the energy of these worlds into your soul also. Perhaps you can see the healing angel Rafael here with his green and purple wings. Stay in this lower world *Yod*. Receive the physical and spiritual vibrations of our universe, within your soul.

9. Now visualize the *Vav* that separates the Lower Worlds and the World

of God. This is like a veil that separates our consciousness from God consciousness. Receive its energy. Visualize its purple energy. This is the energy of Balance, of *Tiferet*, balancing the energies of the Lower Worlds with the energies of the Upper Worlds.

10. Now, float up into the upper *Yod*, the Higher Reality. Visualize it as green and receive its energy. This is the energy of *Nefesh Elohit*, the Celestial World of God, the world of *Atzilut*. Dissolve your "I" into the "Greater I." Become one with the One. Feel completely connected with the One. Feel the consciousness of the Higher *Yod*. Feel your consciousness attach to the Higher Consciousness. The energy of the Lower Worlds and the energy of the Higher Worlds share the same color green, because both are really one. Enjoy feeling connected with the One. Completely receive the energy of the Upper World of *Atzilut,* the world of God Consciousness.

11. When you are ready, float down into the *Vav*. Enjoy receiving the healing purple energy of *Vav*. Then, again when you are ready, float down into the lower *Yod*. See its green color. Know that even though you are in the Lower *Yod*, you are part of the Upper *Yod*.

12. Draw back within your mind from the lower *Yod* and, as you step back, see the whole *Alef.* Meditate on this *Alef*, with its purple *Vav* and two green *Yod*s. Know that it expresses God's Unity and God's balance within you, the only true reality. As you look at it, meditate on the oneness of the spiritual and the physical and know that your consciousness and God consciousness are One.

13. As you visualize the *Alef* in this way — from the outside, as it were, with its diagonal purple *Vav* and two green *Yod*s — know and intuit and feel that your Upper Reality and your Lower Reality are in balance. Remember a healthy person is one whose sense of Divinity and sense of humanity are in balance. When God breathed the breath of life into us, we became both human and divine at the same time. The *Alef* represents this dichotomy within us. Just as Dr. Dresher's *gertel* reminded him that the human being is a channel that unites and separates heaven and earth, the *Alef* reminds us that every one of us is a channel through which the energies of our divinity and our humanity flow in balance.

These two Kabbalistic meditations offer different approaches to achieve soul balance within you. When your human energies and divine energies are in balance within your soul, you are in a state of great health and in a position to deliver healing to others.

Kabbalah strives for balance, not for "perfection" as some philosophers do. The Kabbalist strives to achieve a state of soul balance within him/herself, and between him/herself and God. We want our spiritual energies to be in balance within us, as God's spiritual energies are in balance. Achieving and maintaining this balance is another great secret of Kabbalistic healing.

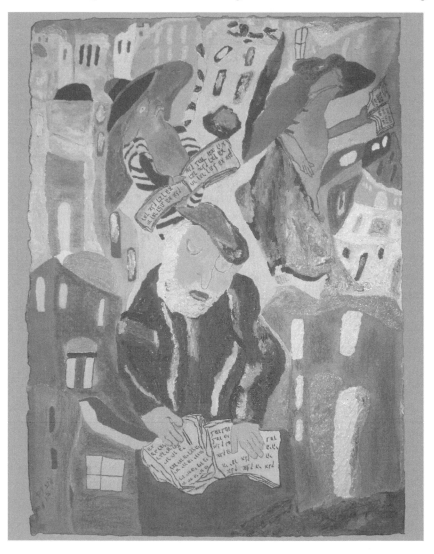

6

The Healing Power of
the Hebrew Letters

WE learn in the oldest Kabbalistic manual, *Sefer Yetzirah,* that God created the Universe using the ten *Sefirot* and the twenty-two Hebrew letters. The *Sefirot* are ten spiritual dimensions that bridge the gap between the physical world and the Divine worlds, including God. These *Sefirot* also exist within God and within us, as *transformers* of divine energy. They also exist as *centers* of energy. Everything is composed of *Sefirot* and the Hebrew letters.

God used twenty-two different *forces* of energy to create the Universe. These different energies are known to us as the letters of the Hebrew alphabet. They originated in the hidden light that God sent into the Universe.

According to Lurianic Kabbalah, in the beginning the *Ayn Sof,* the Infinite as God was called then, was everywhere. The *Ayn Sof* is the source and power of everything. Everything exists because of the *Ayn Sof.* God was, and is, up and down and north and south and east and west.

In his massive work *Etz Chaim*, Rabbi Chaim Vital, Isaac Luria's leading student, teaches that a desire to create the Universe arose within the very center of the *Ayn Sof.* By center, we don't mean a physical center, as the *Ayn Sof* is infinite. Because the *Ayn Sof* was everywhere, there was no room for a universe. So the Infinite God withdrew His light from the center of His being to create a place. He withdrew Himself into Himself. This mystical process of withdrawing Himself into Himself is called *tzimtzum.*

When the *Ayn Sof* did this, He created a place for an *Other* to exist by receiving from Him. The Other, the newly created vacuum, must *receive* from God in order to exist. This empty space was called the *Halal.*

It wasn't completely empty, though, as nothing can be empty of God — there was a residue of God's Light in it. The *Zohar* calls this the *Tehiru ila'ah,* or the Supernal Light. Within this Supernal Light or residue left over from the *tzimtzum,* twenty-two intelligent energy forces came into being.

Please understand that although I use the word "other" here, this "other" is an aspect of God. All separations and all distances from God are from our perception. From God's point of view, all is still One and within Him.

These twenty-two intelligent energy forces are the creative light forces behind everything. They create and sustain the entire universe. They express themselves through the shapes and energies of the Hebrew alphabet. Each Hebrew letter is a different energy force and instrument of power. Their sound and sight vibrations, their physical forms, are the DNA forces of Creation. Various sequences of Hebrew letters release enormous amounts of spiritual energy.

ל	Lamed *has the sound of l*	א	Alef *silent letter*
מ	Mem *has the sound of m*	ב	Bet/Vet *has the sound of b or v*
נ	Nun *has the sound of n*	ג	Gimel *has the sound of g*
ס	Samech *has the sound of s*	ד	Dalet *has the sound of d*
ע	Ayin *silent letter*	ה	Hey *has the sound of h*
פ	Pey/Fey *has the sound of P or F*	ו	Vav *has the sound of v*
צ	Tzadik *has the sound of tz*	ז	Zayin *has the sound of z*
ק	Kuf *has the sound of k*	ח	Chet *has the sound of ch*
ר	Resh *has the sound of r*	ט	Tet *has the sound of t*
ש	Shin/Sin *has the sound of s or sh*	י	Yod *has the sound of y*
ת	Tav *has the sound of t*	כ	Kaph *has the sound of k or kh*

In the alphabets of ordinary language, letters have *representational* power. But in the Hebrew alphabet, letters have *creative* power. When God first created the heavens and the Earth, He not only filled them up with molecules and atoms and quarks but also with Hebrew letters. Every bit of Earth, for example, is made up of the Hebrew letters that make *Adamah*, the word for "Earth" in Hebrew.

God uses thirty-two forces in Creation — the ten *Sefirot* and the twenty-two letters. The ten *Sefirot* are referred to as lights. The twenty-two letters are vessels. The entire world operates through a hidden language, a code based on the Hebrew letters. A Kabbalistic healer is taught how to use these forces in creating health.

The *Sefirot* and the letters correspond meticulously to the different parts of the human body. For example, the letter *Hey* corresponds to the right leg. The letter *Ayin* corresponds to the liver. The letter *Kuf* corresponds to the spleen. *Alef* corresponds to the chest. And so on and so on. Look closely at the Hebrew letters on page 90. Study each one of them. Each of these letters can be meditated upon to bring about miraculous healing. (See page 99 for a chart of all the letters and their corresponding limbs or organs.)

Each organ not only corresponds to a Hebrew letter, it also has a Hebrew name. The heart, for example has the Hebrew name *Lev*, comprised of the letters *Lamed* and *Vet*. In praying for the wellness of the heart, we visualize on the heart the letter *Alef* that corresponds to it, and the letters *Lamed* and *Vet* that make up the Hebrew word for heart.

Every aspect of God's being has a name. God wanted to manifest these Holy names when creating the universe. When certain energy forces are put together in sequential order, the combination brings us face to face with the energy of God.

God's essential name, for example, is *YHVH* יהוה. We believe that these four letters are not representational, but are a *manifestation* of God. This name has its root in the three-letter Hebrew verb *HOVEH* הוה which means to be. When we add *Yod*, the fourth letter, to this verb, we activate and transform it into the future tense or the imperative tense. We see God's essential nature through this name as *active being,* or *being in action.* It can be translated as "He was, He is, He will be." Seeing the Face of God in *YHVH* יהוה is a Kabbalistic secret of healing.

Here are two healing meditations using God's essential name, the name with which He created and still creates this universe. Often when I sit with someone in prayer, we do one of these meditations together — to identify ourselves with the Presence of the Living God. Each of them is very efficacious in bringing about healing. Ideally, I and the person I am praying for both do the meditation. If the other person is in too much pain or is not feeling well, I do it alone, strengthening my identification with *Hashem* so that my prayers for the person will be extra strong.

HOW TO: Healing Meditation #1 Using *YHVH*

Before you begin this meditation, say *Shiviti YHVH l'negdi tamid* שִׁוִּיתִי יְהֹוָה לְנֶגְדִּי תָמִיד five times in Hebrew and one time in English "I place *YHVH* before me always" (Psalm 16:8).

1. Visualize a *Yod* י five inches in front of your forehead, filled with flames — red, orange, and gold flames. It is beautiful. Watch the different colored flames dance in it with joy. As you breathe in through your nostrils, see the flaming *Yod* י move toward your forehead and affix itself to your forehead.

2. As you breathe out through your nostrils, visualize a *Hey* ה being established across your right shoulder, past your left shoulder and down both arms. It is filled with blue flames — dark, medium, and light blue flames. Revel in this *Hey* ה with its many colored blue flames.

3. Now visualize a *Vav* ו about seven inches in front of your solar plexus, from your throat down your torso. It is filled with flames of purple — light and dark purple — and they are jumping for joy. Breathe in through your nostrils and see the *Vav* ו coming within you. The *Vav* ו also establishes itself along the spine. See its purple flames on your spine.

4. As you breathe out, a *Hey* ה is established across your waist and hips, and down your legs. This *Hey* ה is filled with pink fire — light, dark, and medium pink. The flames are dancing.

5. We continue to visualize the *YHVH* יְהוָה in these different colors. We become partners with God in creating health. We have become chariots for God because we have invited God to come and sit and be and mingle with us. As you experience yourself filling with God, you can now make your prayer request of God. Often if I am praying

for someone, whether she has cancer or a very serious skin disease or heart disease, I first employ this meditation to become one with God, and then I offer my prayer to God for her.

HOW TO: Healing Meditation #2 Using *YHVH*

Rabbi Yaakov showed me another way to do this healing meditation with someone who is not well. I was inspired by it right away and continue to use it often.

After I have done the healing prayer meditation above, identifying myself with *Hashem* by using the four holy letters of Creation, I then ask the person I am praying for to stand or sit in front of me. I then gently draw with my index finger the *Yod* י with its many orange, red, and gold colors on her forehead. Then I draw a *Hey* ה with its colored flames of blue across her shoulders and down her arms. Next I draw down her solar plexus, from the throat down through the torso, a *Vav* ו filled with dancing purple flames. I know that this *Vav* also establishes itself down her spine. I then draw a *Hey* ה across her waist and down both legs, filled with many pink flames. Finally, we both hold hands and say together: *I place YHVH before me always. I am created in the Image of God.*

These *YHVH* healing meditations are interactive. When we do them together, I and the person I am praying for both know that we are *activating* the Presence of God within us. Though everyone is *filled* with the Presence of God, not everyone is *activated* with the Presence of God. For healing to begin, one's inner "God Principle" must be activated.

For example, my study in our synagogue is wired for electricity. The ceiling lights are strong and the lamp behind my desk is beautiful. Yet, if I am the first one in my office (which is very rare), my study is completely dark. I need to turn on or activate the electrical current before the lights in my study shine. In the same way, even though God dwells within each one of us — we all are hardwired with God — we need to activate God within us. These special meditations fill us with the Living God. Shining brightly within us, this Living God sets us on our way to healing.

When used properly in meditation, Psalm 16:8 is very powerful in keeping all your *Sefirot* in balance; but Psalm 16:8 also has the amazing ability to identify you with *Hashem* completely. There is an expression *translator traitor*, which means that translation is at best deceptive. This is clearly so in most English translations of the Bible, especially with respect to Psalm 16:8. The English translation usually says *I placed the Presence of the Lord before me,* or *I place the Presence of the Lord before me always,* or *I am ever mindful of the Lord's Presence.* We must stop translating *YHVH* into Lord! The correct usage is "I place *YHVH* before me always." That is, I place the energies of *Yod* and the energies of *Hey* and the energies of *Vav* and the energies of *Hey*, in that sequential order, before me always. I place the Face of God before me always.

The key here is to visualize these four letters, *YHVH*, on your body. When you visualize the Hebrew letters of *YHVH* on your body, you are visualizing God's male energy liberating the *Shechina* or God's female energy *ADNY*. When we liberate *ADNY* from Her exile, we create balance. Then, when you leave your home or do your work, when you pray with people or eat your dinner, you are able to recollect these four letters (that you mentally placed on your body earlier) in the morning as part of your *being*. And remember, these are not really "letters." They are *intelligent energies,* in a *sequential order.* If you recollect them on the different parts of your body, or on your energy centers, whether you are doing a business deal or a healing you will have remarkable results. This is another amazing secret of Kabbalistic healing.

As mentioned earlier, the *Sefer Yetzirah* correlates each Hebrew letter with a different part of the human body. When one does Kabbalistic healing with the Hebrew letters, she meditates on a specific letter that correlates with the limb or organ she is praying for. In doing this, she strengthens the spiritual energy of that limb or organ. As she meditates on the limb and its corresponding Hebrew letter, she focuses her *kavvanah* on that letter and draws spiritual energy and healing power into its corresponding limb or organ. Not only is there a direct correlation between letters and different limbs and organs, there is also a correspondence with the seven openings of the senses of the human body: two eyes, two ears, two nostrils, mouth.

Classical Kabbalists, however, are not all consistent with the particular correlatives of the Hebrew letters. My experience has taught me to choose the system of one Kabbalist only and to use it consistently.

Chapters 2:2 and 6:7 of *Sefer Yetzirah* show us different ways to meditate on the Hebrew letters, each of which has a unique shape, a particular sound, and a corresponding numerical value. It asks us first to choose a letter. For example, a *Bet:* the Torah begins with the letter *Bet* ב. Really *look* at it. See its visual shape. When we feel very comfortable looking at the letter and feel a relationship to it, we are to close our eyes and continue to see it in our mind's eye. Then we are to see this *Bet* in the ten colors of the *Sefirot* — see it first in our mind's eye as translucent gold, then as a white energy force, then as a green energy force, then in baby blue, then in blood red. We are to see it next in purple. Then in light pink, dark pink, orange, and navy blue. This is according to the *Sefirotic* color map Moses Cordovero uses in his book *Pardes Rimonim.*

By gazing at the Hebrew letter in these ten different colors, we access its particular divine energy in the most profound way. I suggest you do with each of the Hebrew letters what we just did with the *Bet.* This is a wonderful way to develop a keen relationship with each of the twenty-two intelligent life-force energies that have corresponding parts of the human body. Visualizing each letter in this way, on its corresponding body part, is an excellent way to initiate great healing.

Sefer Yetzirah 2:2 also suggests that we engrave the Hebrew letter in our mind's eye. When you do this meditation, imagine that you are an artist in an art studio, with an awl or a chisel in your hand, facing a block of marble. Now, in your mind's eye, use your tool to carve the letter *Bet* ב into the stone. When you finish, stare at this *Bet* you have carved in the stone. See it, in sequence, in the *ten energetic colors of the Sefirot*: translucent gold, white, green, baby blue, blood red, purple, light pink, dark pink, orange, and navy blue.

Another meditative technique in *Sefer Yetzirah* 2:2 is to sculpt the letter. In this meditation, you face your block of marble and carve away everything around the letter, until only the letter remains. Then visualize it in the ten energetic colors of the *Sefirot*: translucent gold, white, green, baby blue, blood red, purple, light pink, dark pink, orange, and navy blue.

This technique can be done for each of the twenty-two Hebrew letters.

Here are two other meditative techniques derived from Chapter 2 of *Sefer Yetzirah:*

In the first meditation, close your eyes, and imagine yourself in the center of a circle composed of the twenty-two Hebrew letters. You can be either sitting or standing in your imagination. Visualize each of these letters around you as a three-dimensional form. So you are sitting or standing in the center of a circle made of twenty-two 3-D Hebrew letters. With your mind's eye, scan and see every letter in front of or behind you, until you can see all the letters in front of and behind you at the same time. Visualize each letter filled with flames of red, gold, orange, and blue.

For the second meditation, close your eyes and visualize that you are lying down. Above you on the ceiling are two circles, one within the other. In the outer circle are all twenty-two Hebrew letters in black fire. Within the inner circle, near its edge is the letter *Alef* in white fire. Visualize the outer circle moving clockwise, so that first the *Alef* in black fire aligns above the *Alef* in white fire. Next, the *Bet* in black fire aligns with the *Alef* in white fire, then the *Gimel* in black fire aligns with the *Alef* in white fire. Continue this process with each of the remaining letters. After you finish a complete rotation of the letters, replace the *Alef* on the inner circle with a white *Bet.* Visualize this *Bet* aligned with the *Alef* in black fire, then the *Bet* in black fire, and so on as before. Do this for each of the twenty-two letters of the alphabet, so that each has its turn in the inner circle. This technique is derived from *Mishna* 1:11 and 2:4 of *Sefer Yetzirah.*

———————

These meditations I have just shared are all excellent in helping you become comfortable in your knowledge of the Hebrew letters. Become fluent in one or two, or maybe three. When you are, you will be able to visualize the Hebrew letters corresponding to the parts of the body of the person you are praying for. You will be able to place the appropriate letter on an organ or limb, knowing that its energy is facilitating healing in your prayer partner.

When you feel a relationship and strong connection with each of the Hebrew letters, you can use each one of these intelligent life-energy forces in healing. Recently, for example, I have been praying with several people suffering from hepatitis. The Hebrew letter or energy force that corresponds to the liver is *Ayin*. I visualize the liver with many *Ayin*s on it. I either see them in one color — perhaps purple, the color of healing — or I see them in the ten colors of the *Sefirot*.

The reason a certain letter corresponds with a certain organ or limb is because the life-energy of that letter is the same life-energy that keeps that organ or limb in excellent health. Just as God uses the letters to bring forth energy in Creation, we do the same. We use a specific letter to bring good healing energy to this specific organ.

Here is the letter-healing meditation in full:

HOW TO: Deliver Healing Energy of the Hebrew Letters

1. Sit facing the person you are praying for. Hold hands with one another. If this is not possible, then hold just one of your friend's hands.

2. Breathe in gently through your nostrils, and exhale gently through your nostrils. Do this a few times, aware that you are breathing in God's Presence.

3. Now visualize the *Ayin* ע which correlates to the liver, using any of the Hebrew letter imaging techniques discussed above. When I do this, I use two or three of them one after another. This connects me most strongly with the Hebrew letter I want to use.

4. Visualize a beam of light coming from the heavens, through the roof, onto the crown of your head. This beam of light is filled with many *Ayin*s.

5. As you breathe in through your nostrils, this beam of light filled with *Ayin*s on the crown of your head enters your chest area, filling your chest with light and *Ayin*s. As you breathe out through your nostrils, God's healing light, filled with *Ayin*s, travels through your arms, through the arms of the person you are praying for, and into her liver.

6. Do this five times.

7. Visualize the liver of the person you are praying for, filled with *Ayins* — either in purple or in the ten energetic colors.

8. Ask God to heal the person you are praying for. Ask God to heal her with the faith that, as you are praying, the healing has already begun.

9. Visualize her healed and thank God for healing her.

This prayer meditation can be done with any organ or limb. Consult the table at the end of this chapter to find the appropriate letter for the organ or limb you are praying for. You will notice that the list is not comprehensive. *Sefer Yetzirah* was written thousands of years ago, before we had today's intricate knowledge of our anatomy. When I am praying for an illness, such as diabetes, which is not covered in this chart, I focus on a related location or organ, such as the abdomen, which is where the pancreas is located.

I recognize, as does the Talmud, that it is much more difficult to pray for healing for yourself. I remember the number of times I had surgery in the hospital. Upon awakening, the pain was great but my optimism was not. It was hard to do healing prayer for myself. But, if no prayer partner is available, you can visualize a beam of light from the heavens filled with the energetic letters that are needed to heal the specific organ coming through the roof onto the crown of your head.

As you breathe in, visualize the light being activated and delivering the healing energetic letters to the affected organ. As you breathe out, feel the healing taking place. Do this five times. Ask God in your own words to heal you. Don't be shy. Talk to God as if He is your loving parent. He is. Visualize yourself healed. Thank God from the bottom of your heart for healing you.

The Healing Power of the Hebrew Letters, according to *Sefer Yetzirah*

Letter	Hebrew Letter	Part of Body
Alef	א	Chest
Bet	ב	Right eye
Gimel	ג	Right ear
Dalet	ד	Right nostril
Hey	ה	Right leg
Vav	ו	Right kidney
Zayin	ז	Left leg
Chet	ח	Right hand
Tet	ט	Left kidney
Yod	י	Left hand
Kaph	כ	Left eye
Lamed	ל	Gall bladder
Mem	מ	Abdomen
Nun	נ	Intestines
Samech	ס	Lower bowels
Ayin	ע	Liver
Pey	פ	Left ear
Tzadik	צ	Stomach
Kuf	ק	Spleen
Resh	ר	Left nostril
Shin	ש	Head
Tav	ת	Mouth

In addition to teaching that the twenty-two Hebrew letters are building blocks of creation, *Sefer Yetzirah* teaches that each letter corresponds to a different part of the human body. Meditating on its corresponding Hebrew letter draws healing spiritual energy into that specific area.

The Three H's of Healing

KABBALISTIC healing is *homeopathic, holographic,* and *holistic.* Each of these three qualities involves a mysterious secret.

Like Cures Like

According to conventional sources, homeopathy in its current form was founded by Dr. Samuel Hahnemann (1755–1843) in 1796. It is based on the concept that "like cures like" (the principle of similars) and treats diseases with minute doses of drugs whose effects mimic symptoms of the disease being treated. The idea is that a person's illness can be cured by something that creates the same pattern of symptoms in someone who is well. Some sources trace this idea and practice back to Hippocrates in about 400 BC.

The Kabbalah maintains most clearly that homeopathy, even as we know it today, has its origin in the Torah. The story of the Golden Calf offers a good example of using homeopathic medicine that is recorded in the Bible:

And when the people saw that Moses delayed to come down from the mount, the people gathered themselves unto Aaron and said to him, "Make us a god who shall go before us; for this Moses . . . we know not what has become of him . . . and all the people broke off the golden rings that were in their ears and brought them to Aaron. He received it and fashioned it with an engraving tool and made it a molten calf. And they said "this is thy god O Israel which brought thee out of the land of Egypt." . . . Moses

turned and went down from the mountain with the two tables
of the testimony in his hand. . . . And it came to pass as soon as
he came into the camp, that he saw the calf and the dancing, and
Moses's anger waxed hot and he cast the tablets out of his hands
and broke them beneath the mount and he took the calf which they
had made and burnt it with fire and ground it to powder and he
threw it upon the water and made the children of Israel drink it
(Exodus 32:1–20).

Moses responded to the idolatrous nature of his people by first removing the idol — an object that lacked any spiritual merit — from its exalted
position, and then he brilliantly applied a spiritual homeopathic solution.
He "cured" the people of idolatry by giving them a bit of the idol to
drink. Some people died, but the great majority survived the application
of "like cures like." They would not dare to practice idolatry again. Their
soul illness became soul wellness.

Many years after the incident of the Golden Calf, Moses was faced with
another medical emergency. Again he used the Kabbalistic secret of "like
cures like," albeit in a different way.

And they journeyed from Mt. Hor by way of the Red Sea, to com-
pass the land of Edom; and the soul of the people became impatient,
because of the way. And the people spoke against God and against
Moses. "Why have you brought us up out of Egypt to die in the wilderness? For there is no bread and there is no water; and our soul
loathes this light bread." And the Lord sent fiery serpents among
the people and they bit the people; and many people of Israel died.
So the people came to Moses and said, "We have sinned because we
have spoken against the Lord and against thee; pray unto the Lord
that He take away the serpent from us." And Moses prayed for the
people. And the Lord said to Moses, "Make thee a fiery serpent and
set it upon a pole; and everyone that is bitten, when he sees it, shall
live." Then Moses made a serpent of brass and set it upon the pole;
and it came to pass that if a serpent had bitten any man, when he
looked onto the serpent of brass, he lived (Numbers 21:4-9).

For these poisonous snakebites, God prescribes a cure based on like cures like. Here it's "snake cures snake." The Israelites are cured this time not by swallowing something but by gazing on something. Yet the principle remains: like cures like.

After the splitting of the Red Sea, Moses and the children of Israel traveled in the wilderness for three days and could find no water. When they finally came to a place called Marah, there was water. But the water was very bitter, and the people couldn't drink it. They complained and demanded that Moses offer a solution.

Rabbi Bachya ben Asher, a medieval Jewish mystic, teaches in his mystical commentary to the Torah that when Moses prayed to alleviate the bitterness of the water, God instructed him to sweeten it by throwing a piece of bitter wood into it. God showed Moses again that like cures like.

Rabbi Bachya offers another example of like cures like in Kings 2:20, which says: "Bring me a new dish and put salt in it." Here, Elisha salts the water. Instead of making the water even less palatable, as we would expect, adding a little salt turns it into drinking water. Like cures like.

The Tzemach Tzedek, the third Lubavitcher Rebbe, teaches that God wounds and heals with the same medium. We see this in Scripture again and again. Within every human being, there is a unique spiritual force which maintains and vitalizes the body at all times. This force responds vigorously and positively to homeopathic methods, which appear to be a preferred method of healing by God.

Holographic Healing

In modern western medicine, it is crucial to understand mathematics. A comprehensive grasp of logic is equally important. For these reasons and these reasons alone, as a sixteen-year-old high school student from Montreal, Quebec, I was unable to apply to medical school. I stunk at math and was even worse in the study of logic. My very expensive high school math tutors would say, "Why can't you get it? If $A = B$, and $B = C$, then $A = C$." I probably did get that simple logical equation, but only with a great deal of effort. The more difficult logical equations flew over my head, and there went medical school.

But if I had been born twenty years later, I could have been a doctor *and* a rabbi, thanks to a relatively new branch of mathematics called "fuzzy logic." Not only do I understand fuzzy logic, I *qvell* when I am faced with problems that involve using fuzzy logic. *Qvell* is Yiddish for your whole body tingling with pride and joy from head to toe.

Kabbalah is clear that the nature of manifest reality has changed enormously over the years. In the beginning, we were "thought forms" mingling with one another on a spiritual plane of existence. We were all one grand soul. This doesn't deny that we were unique beings, yet we were also all connected with one another and with God. Then came Adam and Eve's sin of wrong eating and the collapse into a physical world. Our reality changed from a spiritual universe to the physical universe in which we live. Because of this, we face tremendously ambiguous urges — including the urge to go back to the good old days when we were all connected. It is likely that these urges are what inspire us to participate daily in Facebook: we have a distant memory of all being One.

So our Reality is ambiguous — especially as we learn from Kabbalah that there is more than this physical universe and that we live in parallel universes, or realms. The Divine realm is the world of *Atzilut.* The realm of Mind is called *Briah,* or Creation. The realm of Emotion is called *Yetzirah,* or the world of Formation. *Assiyah,* this physical world, is the world of time and space and earthly consciousness. So you see, we really do experience the nature of reality ambiguously. And Fuzzy Logic reflects this new reality.

With classical logic, answers are either yes or no. Fuzzy Logic embraces nuance, such as in dealing with the statement that there are more Protestants than Jews. This is true and false. It's true overall, but there are exceptions to the general rule. There are many places where there are more Jews than Protestants, and I don't mean only in Israel.

Kabbalah embraces fuzzy logic because Kabbalah embraces a holographic world model. In a holographic system every part not only contains information about itself, it also contains information about every other part in the system. A holographic universe is one in which each part of the universe has within itself a form of every other part of the Universe — in everything is everything.

The Principle of Inter-inclusion

Lurianic Kabbalah maintains that every human being, every fox, every mountain, every thing, is made up of ten *Sefirot*. Gershom Scholem, in his book *Kabbalah*, maintains that "The *Sefirot* both individually and collectively subsume the archetype of every created thing. Just as they are contained in the Godhead, so they impregnate every being outside it."[1] The ten *Sefirot* are spiritual dimensions which bridge the gap between the physical world and the Divine world. They exist also within us, as energy centers and transformers of energy.

In the diagram called the Tree of Life, the *Sefirot* are arranged in triads that resemble three columns, as shown at right. The right column — *Chochma, Chesed, Netzach* — represents God's love and kindness. The left column — *Bina, Gevurah, Hod* — represents Judgment and the Power of Restraint. The middle column — *Keter, Tiferet, Yesod, Malchut* — represents Mercy and the balance of Love and Restraint.

The right column represents the ability to give. The left represents the ability to receive, or to hold back from giving. The middle represents arriving at a balance between giving and holding back. Even though right/giving and left/restraint are diametrically opposed, Luria maintains that if these two concepts were not *inter-inclusive*, if each didn't contain its own opposite within itself, the two would never be able to interact, to give birth, to produce. The right and left columns of the Tree of Life are therefore necessarily inter-inclusive and holographic, demonstrating the Kabbalistic principle of Inter-inclusion. God is One. His creation reflects His Oneness in the fact that all opposites — right/left, giving/restraint, male/female — are inter-inclusive.

Since everything is composed of ten *Sefirot* and every *Sefira* is contained within every other *Sefira*, a black-and-white statement about A as opposed to B is never perfectly true Kabbalistically. Since B also contains A, any statement concerning A is also partially true about B. That's why we can't have a Kabbalistic statement that is absolutely and perfectly true. There is always another perspective that offers another interpretation. Things may be true in one context and not have the same truth value in another context. We can, however, make statements that are generally true. For example,

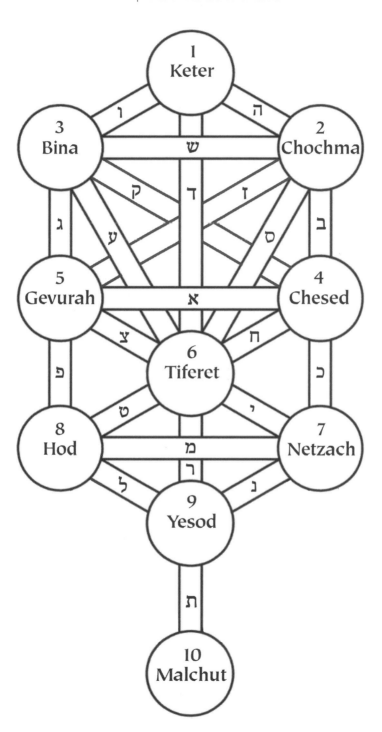

we say that dogs are usually bigger than cats. A Kabbalist remembers constantly that the world is a fuzzy place and its truth, though revered and respected, can be very fuzzy.

Our universe is distinguished by its holographic structure and features. Every piece of it contains every other piece inside itself. Every good contains a bit of evil, and every evil contains a bit of good. Every Jew contains aspects of every non-Jew, every non-Jew contains aspects of Jews. Every man contains aspects of woman, every woman contains aspects of man. Everything is in everything. If there is an illusion that must be dispelled, it is the illusion of "other than God."

So often, people innocently maintain that evil is the opposite of God. There is God. There is Auschwitz. People maintain these are opposites. I recently officiated at the funeral of a young man, for example, who was one of the finest people you could ever know. He died from a virulent form of cancer. His wife had died fifteen years earlier and so his two children left behind are now orphans. I can't tell you how many times I have heard, "Cancer is the devil." There is cancer, and there is God. Two opposites, fighting for control. "Rabbi, evil is so awful. Evil is the opposite of God. Why does God allow this?"

Kabbalah teaches that evil is not the opposite of God. What we call evil is a manifestation of God. God is everything, according to Kabbalah. Good and evil, black and white, illness and wellness, are all manifestations of God. We may ask, "Why does God allow evil to exist? Why does God allow a child to die of leukemia? Why did God allow the Holocaust to happen? Why does God allow people in African nations to starve while people in Western nations embrace riches beyond measure? Why does God allow horrific illnesses to overtake so many of us? Why did God allow two beautiful children to become orphans?"

Kabbalah maintains it is not a matter of purpose and allowing. It's a matter of the unconditional nature of God's *Shlemut*, God's Perfection. If God is God, if God is complete Balance, then God must contain all possibilities. Everything and its opposite. Good and evil are but two of the infinite possibilities of God.

No matter how small the pebble on the beach is, one day, with the right microscope, looking at that pebble, we will be able to understand the structure of the universe. We buy bigger and bigger telescopes to understand the outer universe. Mistake. We need to buy better and better "micro" scopes to understand the human being, as each of us is a true microcosm of the macrocosm. In everything is everything. This is the principle of Inter-inclusion. The world, and each one of us, is holographic. This is another great secret of Kabbalistic healing.

Holistic Healing

The Kabbalah teaches that God, as the all-encompassing principle of existence, has both a male and a female expression. The male aspect is called The Holy One, blessed be He, Father. The female is called the *Shechina*, Mother. The great Kabbalist Rav Tzadok HaKohen writes, in *Dober Tzedik* 2a & 2b, that the essential light of God is so strong and intense that it cannot be grasped or even internalized by the human heart. That's why the Torah says about God, "No one can see My face and live" (Exodus 33:20).

But because God wants to be in relationship with us He contracts and constricts His light so that it dwells within each of us. This aspect of Divinity is called the *Shechina*, which means precisely In-dwelling Presence. God as *Shechina* loves us enormously. That is why, as *Shechina* dwells within each one of us, She gently and constantly raises each of us to our higher destiny. When we recognize that the Presence of God is within us, from head to toe, we are in the Greater Mind. We are in Greater Consciousness. When we deny Her complete Presence within us, we live in a constricted consciousness or Lesser Mind.

Rabbi Tzadok HaKohen has given us a meditation to recognize and embrace the Greater Mind. A person should reflect on the Divine Soul, the *Shechina, Nefesh Elohit,* that exists within, and recognize that this soul is connected to the very Source of Life that fills and surrounds all worlds, the Holy One blessed be He. The *Shechina* dwells within you. This realization, that a piece of God is actually present within one's soul, is so amazing that a person should be in awe and in love when he thinks of it.

In Talmud *Tractate Sanhedrin* 46a, Rabbi Meir teaches that when a person is in pain, the *Shechina* within us is what is saying, "My head aches, my arm aches." Kabbalist Rabbi Chaim of Volozhin interprets this text

Kabbalistically in his masterful treatise, *Nefesh HaChayim* 2:11. He says this Talmudic passage means that when we realize God's pain concerning our illness is even greater than our own, that is the turning point in healing. That we humans, so beloved to Her, suffer in a world that God meant to be perfect, causes tremendous pain to God. She, the *Shechina*, experiences Divine Agony. When we recognize that God's pain is even greater than our own and begin to pray for the *Shechina*, this is the beginning of the end of our suffering. Projecting our care and concern and suffering onto the *Shechina* and allowing ourselves to be involved with the *Shechina is the very essence of Kabbalistic healing.* The Baal Shem Tov teaches that if we can identify and connect with God's Presence inside the pain or suffering or illness, the pain, suffering, illness will go away.

Rabbi Chaim of Volozhin says that when one prays for the relief of the pain of the *Shechina*, one is praying also for the relief of that pain in all who suffer what one suffers, since the *Shechina* dwells in each place of such pain. This is a profound secret of Kabbalistic healing.

When a person is ill, that person feels just like the *Shechina* feels, who is said to be *dala va'aniya* — needy and poor. If you focus on how the *Shechina* suffers, together with all those who suffer your pain, if you identify your personal pain with Hers, you are understanding that we are all connected by and in the *Shechina*. See all those who suffer serious illness as one group and pray for the well-being of all who are afflicted with that suffering. In this way, you embrace a profound secret, and you become a vessel drawing in divine light for yourself as well as for those around you.

When you pray for others, you diminish the severity of the disease not only for yourself, but for others as well. When you think and honestly pray for the *Shechina*, remembering that She suffers not only *your* disease, but She suffers *all* disease, you become a holy vessel, filling up with Divine Light for yourself and for others. You not only receive healing, but you become a healer.

When we wrongfully "own" our disease, we are unwilling to share it with others in our prayers. We may become angry, frustrated, more angry, more upset and resentful. Our suffering will increase. We are unwilling to acknowledge that the *Shechina* within us also suffers. To diminish our suffering, we must project our care, our concern, and our pain onto the

Shechina, recognizing that She is also suffering. To be involved with the *Shechina* this way is a perfect example of the Kabbalistic secret, "Let go and let God."

Here is a meditation that I often do with people who come to pray for healing.

As discussed in our Preface, the *Shechina* is in exile within us — to the extent that our desires, emotions, minds, and souls are constricted because of illness and pain, and we are unable to sense *YHVH* in our lives. To activate the healing principle within each one of us, we need to elevate the *Shechina* and restore Her from Her exile. We need to ask God our Father, *YHVH*, to come down and join with Her within us. We need to create a balance of the feminine and masculine divine energies within us if we want healing.

יהוה YHVH

אדני ADONAI

יאהדונהי – combination of YHVH and ADONAI

HOW TO: A Holistic Meditation that Restores and Returns the *Shechina* from Her Exile

1. Sit down in your *mi'at meekdash*. Unbuckle your belt and be aware of your natural breathing.

2. Focus on your breathing and block out external stimuli from the physical senses. See yourself as separate from every other thing in the room. See the "I" within you as separate from the "not-I's" outside of you. This "I" within is the *Shechina*, or *Adonai*. As you focus on and recognize this "I" within, you are beginning to liberate the "I" within from exile.

3. Visualize the letter energies of *Adonai* אדני in green characters in every cell of your diseased or injured organ or limb. As you recognize the "I" within and visualize the energies of *Adonai* אדני within every injured cell, you are allowing yourself to be open to the large "I" or *YHVH* יהוה which is transcendent to yourself.

4. Visualize *YHVH* יהוה, God Transcendent, about eight inches in front of you in large purple letters. Recognize that this *YHVH* is

symbolic of the infinite *YHVH* that exists in all directions outside of you — north, south, east, west, up and down.

5. When you have liberated *Adonai* from exile by recognizing the little "I" within or *Adonai* in every cell in step 3, and are aware of the presence of God Transcendent in step 4, it is time to end the exile of the *Shechina* from Her Male Consort. It is time to bring *HaKodesh Barchu* or *Hashem* within you, and connect it to *Shechina*, to elevate Her to God Transcendent. We do this by simultaneously: visualizing *Adonai* אדני in green characters (as in step 3); visualizing *YHVH* יהוה in purple letters (as in step 4), and then ending the exile by putting the *Shechina* back together with God Transcendent. To end the exile, bring the letters of *Adonai* and *YHVH* together — visualize יאהדונהי in alternating green and purple characters about eight inches in front of you.

6. Now visualize this יאהדונהי in green and purple characters in every cell in your body.

7. Know that every cell now has male and female divine energies in balance. Every cell is healthy. See yourself well and thank God for healing you.

HOW TO: Loving the Lord Healing Meditation (with another person)

1. Go to your *mi'at meekdash*. You and your friend should both be dressed comfortably. Sit opposite your friend. You the healer are sitting in one seat and your ill friend is sitting in another seat, facing you, and if possible, you are both holding hands.

2. Visualize, with your eyes closed, a beam of light coming down from the heavens, through the roof, onto the crown of your head (*Keter*).

3. Inhale gently and deeply through your nostrils. At the same time, activate the beam of light so that, when you breathe in, the light is activated and travels through *Keter* into your heart (*Tiferet*).

4. Hold your breath for 3–4 seconds and see your heart fill with gold/white light/energy.

5. As you breathe out through your nostrils, you silently say, *You shall love the Lord your God with all your heart, with all your soul, and with all your might.* When you say the word "heart," visualize your heart opening up and the gold/white healing light/energy flowing

from your heart, through the air, into your friend, filling every single cell of her or his body with gold/white healing light/energy. See or feel every cell in your friend's body — every cell — receiving healing light/energy. View yourself as a vessel of *divine healing energy*. Do this for several minutes. It is important that you actually feel you are God's conduit delivering the Transcendent energy into your friend's cells.

6. Now visualize again the beam of light coming down from the heavens, through the roof onto *Keter,* your crown, but this time see the beam of light filled with millions of sets of purple YHVHs יהוה, representing the Holy One Blessed be He, Father.

7. As in step 3, gently breathe in through your nostrils. This time, as you breathe in, visualize gold/white healing light/energy, filled with millions of purple sets of *YHVH* יהוה, moving down through *Keter* into *Tiferet,* at your heart area.

8. Hold your breath for 3–4 seconds, and see your heart fill with divine light/energy, filled with millions of purple *YHVHs* יהוה.

9. As you exhale through your nostrils, say to yourself, "You shall love the Lord your God with all your heart, with all your soul, and with all your might." When you say "heart," again visualize your heart opening up — and this time, visualize gold/white light/energy filled with sets of purple *YHVHs* יהוה flowing from your heart into your friend. Know that every diseased cell of the afflicted organ is being transformed to a *healthy cell* by the joining of *YHVH* with millions of sets of green *Adonai* אדני, which are already within your friend's body. Visualize יאהדונהי on the organ in alternating green and purple characters. Know you have elevated the *Shechina* to God Transcendent. You have ended Her exile. Feel confident that healing is taking place. See the affected organ filled with healing gold/white light energy and know that you are the vessel of divine healing energy from God.

10. Repeat steps 7–9. This time when you get to the stage where you visualize your friend's affected organ as filled with sets of purple *YHVHs* יהוה, also see the whole organ filled with shining light. Then again see on it the letters *YHVH* יהוה joining/merging with the already existing letters of *Adonai* אדני — so that in each cell of it you are now visualizing *YAHDVNHY* יאהדונהי. Each of these

Holy Letters is a powerful form of divine energy — and when they are written in this sequence, the combined energy is truly amazing.

13. After seeing *YAHDVNHY* יאהדונהי on the organ, as you hold your friend's hands with love, think how much you love her or him, and know also that God lives in your friend. Ask God to heal your friend's affected organ. Tell God how much you love your friend, and how good your friend is, and why she or he should be healed. Remember that God lives in your friend.

14. Then visualize your friend completely well. Remember, when you pray, you pray as if your prayer is already answered. See her doing an activity she couldn't do when she was ill. And thank God for having healed her.

HOW TO: Holistic Prayer for Healing, Identifying Your Personal Pain with the *Shechina*

The Talmud recognizes that in a majority of times, we need someone to pray for us when we ourselves are in great pain. It is very difficult for the prisoner to release himself from prison without assistance, as we see on page 175 in the Talmudic story of Rabbi Yochanan. However, Dr. Dan Dresher shared with me a healing meditation that one can do alone in private, based on holistic principles.

When you focus on how the *Shechina* suffers together with all those who suffer your illness, and when you identify your personal pain with the *Shechina*, you are no longer alone.

1. Go to your *mi'at meekdash* and sit on a comfortable chair with your back upright and your feet planted firmly on the floor. Wear comfortable clothing and loosen your tie or belt.

2. Breathe in and out through your nostrils deeply and gently, in a relaxed way.

3. Close your eyes. Visualize *YHVH* יהוה in purple characters about eight inches in front of you.

4. Feel the pain and discomfort in your affected organ, or wherever the pain is in your body.

5. With your eyes still closed, visualize *YHVH* יהוה in purple characters about eight inches in front of you. Recognize that there are

thousands of other people whose *Shechina* experiences this same pain in the same place and with the same intensity.

6. As you continue to visualize *YHVH* יהוה in purple characters, know that God's *Shechina* is within you. Know that not only is She experiencing your pain, She is also experiencing the pain of everyone who suffers the same condition that you do.

7. Continue to visualize *YHVH* יהוה in purple characters in front of you.

8. Visualize the many people who are suffering your disease, each person filled with *Shechina,* each person filled with cells of *Adonai* אדני in green characters.

9. Feel the suffering of all these people together which is the *Shechina* within them, because she has not been liberated.

10. Pray from your heart for the well-being of all those who are afflicted with your disease, and visualize the cells of each person in all this collection of people filled with *Adonai* אדני in green characters. Know that the *Shechina* is in every one of them and She also suffers. As you pray for them all collectively, you pray for the *Shechina* in everyone.

11. Know that as you do this you become a vessel, drawing in divine light for yourself and for all those afflicted with this disease. With your eyes closed, visualize the elevation of *Adonai/Shechina,* joining God the Father, God Transcendent *YHVH* יהוה, in purple characters, now activated within you, since you have prayed for the collective and for the *Shechina*. Visualize *YAHDVNHY* יאהדונהי in alternating colors of green and purple. See yourself well and thank God. Know that everyone who suffers your condition has יאהדונהי energies in their cells.

12. Know that the *Shechina* has been restored from Her exile in everyone who suffers from your condition. When you pray with the knowledge that you are also praying for the *Shechina* and for all those who have your disease, you *automatically* become a vessel that brings down divine healing from *Hashem*. Know that you are completely well and thank *Hashem* for your healing.

HOW TO: Holistic Prayer for Healing with Extra Voltage

1. Repeat steps 1 and 2 above.

3. Close your eyes. Visualize *Adonai* אדני in green characters on the organ that is injured or hurt.

4. Feel the pain and discomfort in your affected organ, or wherever the pain is in your body.

5. Focus on how the *Shechina* also suffers your pain and the pain of all those who suffer your same condition. Identify your personal pain with Hers. Know how She suffers not only your condition but also the condition of all others who suffer as you do.

6. Pray from your heart for the well-being of all those who are suffering with your problem.

7. As you pray, see that you are becoming a vessel, drawing in God's divine transcendent healing light *YHVH* יהוה in purple. This transcendent light joins with the *Shechina* within you to bring Her healing and to bring you healing. With your eyes closed, visualize on the affected organ *YAHDVNHY* יאהדונהי in purple and green.

8. See yourself well and thank God for your healing.

9. Remember that when you identify with the *Shechina*, when you focus on how the *Shechina* suffers with you and with all those who suffer what you suffer, and when you pray for the well-being of others who are afflicted with your same condition, you automatically become a vessel drawing in God's transcendent healing light. You assist in the healing of your affliction by joining together the male and female principles of the Divine, which you can do by visualizing within you, or within your afflicted part: *YAHDVNHY* יאהדונהי.

NOTE

1. Gershom Scholem, *Kabbalah* (Jerusalem: Keter Publishing, 1974) p. 105.

8

The Somersaulting Rabbi

W HO are you? You have a name. You are a female or a male. You have a family. You're a plumber, a doctor, or a lawyer. Does this truly define you?

In Kabbalah, when we ask, "Who are you?" or "Who am I?" we are looking to our *spiritual* center. We call this spiritual center the *Neshamah*. The *Neshamah* is the spiritual umbilical cord that connects you to God. It is the life force that animates you. We could call it the soul, but it is not soul in the same sense as Christians use the word.

For Kabbalists, each person's soul spans and transcends five parallel realms known as *olamot*, worlds. These worlds are not places where creatures inhabit a particular space; rather, they are states of consciousness. Being in a certain world means being in a certain conscious state. The highest world is called *Adam Kadmon* which, as mentioned in Chapter 1, is an intermediate world between the four lower worlds and *Ayn Sof*. This world is the source or the point of communion with the transcendent God we call *Hashem*.

Though I use the words "upper" and "lower," "above" "and below" in describing these states of consciousness, please understand that I am only speaking in terms of their logical priority. The worlds are actually parallel.

The next world, in descending order, is *Atzilut*. This is the Godly Realm, the hidden reality in which everything originates and from which everything emanates. Next is *Briah*, the Soul Realm, the world of Souls. It is the world of Creation, the world of thought. Then we have the world of *Yetzirah*, the Angelic world, the world of Formation, of speech. Last in this order is *Assiyah* the Physical world in which we live, the world of action. So we have:

> *Adam Kadmon*
> *Atzilut* the World of Emanation,
> *Briah* the world of Creation,
> *Yetzirah* the world of Formation,
> *Assiyah* the world of Action.

Each of these parallel worlds manifests key levels of divine energy — thought energies, sound energies, speech energies, and so on. Every person's soul connects with all of them. Every individual soul has energy vibrations that are related to these five worlds. If the energy vibrations of our soul within all these worlds are in balance, we can transfer the vibrations of our soul onto another person.

Only if you have what my *zaidie* [grandfather] called soul balance, or soul muscle, can you offer spiritual and physical healing to another in the best possible way. So this chapter shares more spiritual techniques that help create soul balance.

My grandfather, Rabbi Sheinman, always taught me that a healthy soul leads to a healthy body. A healthy soul creates a healthy body. Our soul and our body are one.

When I was a little boy, about nine or ten, I was teased in school because of the radiation burns on my left hand. My *zaidie* would say again and again how important it is to find that which is special in me and make it shine in the world. One of his favorite rabbis was Rabbi Kalonymus Kalman Shapira, called by his followers the Rebbe of Peasetzna. My *zaidie* loved to quote and talk about this remarkable man, who wrote beautiful commentaries on the Torah in Hebrew which I now regularly study with my seminary students. He was a favorite of my grandfather's and, to my enormous surprise, he also was one of Rabbi Yaakov's favorite teachers and spiritual leaders.

A number of years ago, there was a little boy named Shelly in our congregation. Shelly was the best eight-year-old juggler I had ever seen. He could do with five tennis balls what McEnroe could do with one. I'm exaggerating a bit, but you get the idea. Unfortunately, Shelly often missed Sunday school due to recurrent bouts with fevers. One day he told me that he loved our private study Torah sessions on Wednesday afternoons, but he hated Sunday school because he was the shortest in the class.

One Saturday morning, while we were marching with the Torah around the sanctuary, as is our custom before reading from it in the course of a service, I saw Shelly holding his juggling balls. My instinct was not to ask him to leave the sanctuary, but rather to ask him to march in the procession with the *Sifrei* Torah,[1] while juggling five tennis balls. Was he in his element! He instantly became the synagogue star. It was as if he were the man in the Baal Shem Tov story who throws the Hebrew letters up in the air so that God could form his prayers. When he approached the *bima*, the dais from which we read the Torah in the sanctuary, I asked him to continue juggling on the *bima* as we returned the *Sifrei* Torah to the Ark and undressed the Torah for the morning's reading.

I can't deny that some people were upset that I allowed a little boy to juggle balls on the holy dais. But most people, including his classmates, thought, "Wow! Shelly is cool. Shelly is amazing. We didn't know he could do that." Subsequently, every Shabbat, when we marched with the *Sifrei* Torah, Shelly marched in the procession, juggling tennis balls. All the kids loved it. It brought enormous joy, *Ru'ach*, and *kavvanah* to the *shul* or congregation. Most importantly, Shelly never had a bout with the "flu" again.

When I first saw Shelly juggle and saw how much joy it gave him, I thought of the Rebbe of Peasetzna, or as he was called by many, the Somersaulting Rabbi. The Jewish holiday Simchat Torah — Rejoicing in the Torah — celebrates the conclusion and recommencement of the annual cycle of our reading of the Torah. Traditional synagogues read the Torah every Monday, Thursday, and Saturday morning; Reform synagogues also read the Torah on Friday night. On Simchat Torah, we conclude reading the Five Books of Moses, the Torah, and then begin reading it at the beginning again. We read the last chapter of Deuteronomy and the first chapter of Genesis. It is a tremendous celebration. Jewish people who rarely ever walk into a synagogue dance in the sanctuary with flags and song, apples, and, of course, the *Sifrei* Torah. The singing goes on for hours. In the old Soviet Union, where it was prohibited to practice Torah Judaism, Jews still crowded the streets and thousands and thousands of Jews sang Jewish songs on the streets of Moscow on Simchat Torah.

Rabbi Kalonymus Kalman Shapira was among those who used to march in the procession on *Simchat Torah*. My *zaidie* had heard rumors that Rebbe Shapira also did somersaults every Shabbat when the men marched with the Torah. I asked Rabbi Yaakov if this were true and he said, "Of course; that's why he's called the Somersaulting Rabbi. He always told his parishioners and students that every person must look for his own niche in life. Every person must create his own way. Every person must let his soul shine because, if our soul shines with pride and joy, our bodies will be healthy and strong."

The somersaulting rabbi, through his simple somersaults, taught his students the Kabbalistic secret of holistic healing. He recognized that soul and body are not two, but one. He embraced the Kabbalistic idea that the soul is not limited to being only a treasured divine spark hidden deep in a secret place in our bodies.

I've had children ask, "Is the soul a divine spark hidden in our heart? Is it in our brain? Is it in our liver?" I answer that the soul is everywhere throughout our bodies. As a matter of fact, the Biblical author identified *Nefesh*, or Vital Soul, with the blood of an individual; just as the blood flows throughout the body, so does the soul. The Kabbalah maintains that *Nefesh* is the most fundamental aspect of our soul. It is not only the animating force of animals, but also of inanimate Nature; rivers and trees have *Nefesh*. Throughout our lives, we have the opportunity through good deeds and prayer to activate our *Nefesh* soul so that it reaches higher levels, the levels of *Ru'ach* and *Neshamah*.

We also can tap into the two higher levels of soul, *Chaya* and *Yechidah*, through scrupulously righteous behavior and prayer. They remain in the upper celestial realms, though, and hover over each of us.

The somersaulting rabbi recognized and embraced the holistic nature of Judaism. He knew that a healthy soul, a joyous soul, reflects a healthy and joyous body. He recognized that if a person manifests what is unique to him or her, and embraces this regularly, it leads to physical good health. As the leading rabbi of the Warsaw Ghetto, Rabbi Shapira ministered to thousands and thousands of prisoners in the concentration camps. He needed to be strong and healthy both physically and mentally. And he knew that if he exercised his soul regularly, by bringing out what was unique to him, it would manifest a healthy body.

That is exactly what happened with Shelly. At first, he was short and depressed. But when he became the synagogue juggler, though he remained short, he overcame his flu and depression.

Let's now look closely into the Law of Sympathetic Vibration. This amazing secret of Kabbalistic healing is what reveals that beings attuned to the same frequency can automatically transfer their vibrations from one person to another. According to this law, every person can affect every other person with his/her spiritual vibrations, because each one of us is made up of energies from each of the parallel worlds. But as mentioned above, to do this effectively, the soul and body of the person doing the transferring have to be in balance.

The somersaulting rabbi is an inspiring example of one who understood this principle. He did everything he could to exercise his soul so that the Law of Sympathetic Vibration could manifest powerfully in the wartime Warsaw Ghetto, and the results were truly amazing. One would think that being bombarded by bullets and bombs, the Ghetto citizens would cower and flee from one another, let alone the Nazis. Yet, instead, each Jew fought a private war against his *Yetzer Hara*, evil inclination, and sought to manifest what was uniquely good in him- or herself.

We humans live physically in the time, space, and consciousness of the world of *Assiyah*. Each of us is also necessarily connected to God through the umbilical cord that traverses from *Adam Kadmon*, or *Ayn Sof*, through the worlds, connecting us here with them. When we study Kabbalistic "soul anatomy," we see that even though the Soul is one unit attached to the One God through an umbilical cord of worlds, each human soul has the potential to manifest itself in five ways or levels:

Nefesh	the indwelling soul, common to all life-forms
Ru'ach	Spirit
Neshamah	Divine Soul
Chaya	Living Essence
Yechida	Unique Essence

A person is born with *Nefesh*, the grade of soul which is the raw vital energy necessary for maintaining the engine of the body. The other grades are not achieved until the individual soul has developed soul muscle. The first three of the five, beginning with *Nefesh,* are contained within the body, while the two most developed aspects hover outside the body.

The base of operations of *Nefesh,* or Vital Soul, is the liver and blood. The base of operations of *Ru'ach* is the heart. *Ru'ach* is also located in the medium of breath. *Nefesh* relates to the world of *Assiyah. Ru'ach* relates to the world of *Yetzirah.* The *Neshamah* aspect of soul, our intellectual soul, has its base of operations in the brain. The *Nefesh* level of soul awareness operates when we focus completely on our personal self-concerns. We recognize *Hashem* from our *Nefesh,* from the bottom up.

The *Neshamah* is our direct connection with God — a channel that connects us with God from God down. It is connected to the realm of *Briah,* and has its base of operations in the ears and hearing in addition to the brain. *Chaya* or Life Force is related to *Atzilut. Yechida,* or "Bit of God," is related to *Adam Kadmon.*

The more muscle the soul develops, the more pure it becomes. When it reaches and embraces the stage of *Yechida* awareness, it is so strong that it is offered eternal life, or what we call heaven. An individual soul has many opportunities through *gilgul* — reincarnation or transmigration — to attain this.

Each of these five levels is composed of ten *Sefirot.* Each organ in every human being is likewise composed of ten *Sefirot.* When we are born, we are hardwired to manifest this divine energy in these ten different ways. Without these centers and transformers, we would explode when receiving the Divine Presence, we wouldn't have a surge protector, as it were.

As we studied in Chapter 7, Kabbalah is holistic and holographic. In everything there is everything else. For example, the first of the *Sefirot* is called *Keter,* located on the crown of the head. It is where the umbilical cord connects from *Assiyah* and travels through all the worlds to God. *Keter* receives God's energy and immediately transforms it into an energy that we can maintain. The dominant energy in this energy-transforming center is *Keter* energy. But, holographically, the other nine energies are also present in *Keter.* This holographic pattern applies to every *Sefira* in the body, as to everything in the Universe. The Hebrew word *Sefirot* is a plural; its singular is *Sefira.*

Make Yourself a Chariot for G–d

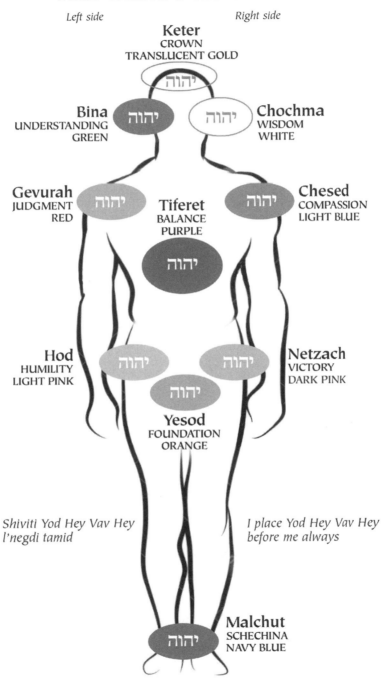

Left side   *Right side*

Keter
CROWN
TRANSLUCENT GOLD

Bina
UNDERSTANDING
GREEN

Chochma
WISDOM
WHITE

Gevurah
JUDGMENT
RED

Tiferet
BALANCE
PURPLE

Chesed
COMPASSION
LIGHT BLUE

Hod
HUMILITY
LIGHT PINK

Netzach
VICTORY
DARK PINK

Yesod
FOUNDATION
ORANGE

*Shiviti Yod Hey Vav Hey
l'negdi tamid*

*I place Yod Hey Vav Hey
before me always*

Malchut
SCHECHINA
NAVY BLUE

Diagram reproduced by permission of Cynthia Dodick

We can map the *Sefirot* on the human body as in the figure at right.

What I've just said about this pattern in *Keter* is true for each *Sefira*. Even though the right shoulder, for example, represents the transformer of divine energy into *Chesed*, Compassion, this same right shoulder contains within itself all the other nine transformers of divine energy. We can bring about healing by activating these transformers of energy, in a balanced way, through meditative practice.

The Chariot for G-d diagram maps the Tree of Life on an outline of the human body. This illustrates the Tree where spiritual and physical are fully integrated. It shows that that not only are soul and body one, but all of us — everything — is one in God. We are all one, as God is One.

The Tree of Life is constant, unified. There is no internal split in the Tree of Life. The Tree of the Knowledge of Good and Evil, in contrast, introduces us to an internal split or dichotomy. When Adam focused on the Tree of Knowledge of Good and Evil, he embraced a split in the Divine, which rejected the Divine Unity of the Tree of Life. This is why Adam and Eve were warned not to eat from the Tree of Knowledge.

When we do healing work, we need to align the Tree of Life with our body as the Chariot diagram shows. The right side of the Tree corresponds to our right brain, our right arm, and right leg. The left side corresponds to our left brain, left arm, and left leg.

Notice that *Keter* covers the crown of the head, while *Chochma* and *Bina* are placed on the right and left sides of the head or brain, respectively. The Crown represents the highest Divinity. This is the crown to your kingdom, which is your body and soul. God's divine energy meets the human here through the transformer of *Keter*. The *Sefira* of *Chochma*, Intuitive Wisdom, represents the Intuitive Mind, the ability to transform the energy of God into intuitive energy. On the left brain we see *Bina*, which means Understanding. This center transforms God's energy into rational energy.

Looking further at our diagram, we arrive at *Chesed*, Compassion. *Chesed* is the energy of Compassion, a transformer of God's energy to compassionate human energy. It originates at the right shoulder, goes down the right arm, and connects to the left shoulder energy called *Gevurah* or *Din:* Severity or Restraint or Judgment. Each of the *Sefirotic* energies has many different names, and each name adds something to our understanding of them.

The name of the energy center called *Tiferet,* which is between *Din* and *Chesed,* can be translated as Harmony or Mercy or Harmonious Energy. Here's an example of how it works. I was recently in downtown Chicago during one of our hottest summers on record. The temperature was over 100° for several days in a row. A homeless man approached me and asked if I could give him forty dollars to cover the expense of a few nights' shelter from the heat. I had no difficulty giving him the money — it was in my pocket and, at that moment, he needed it more than I did. This was an act of *Tiferet* or Harmonious Energy.

After I gave him the forty dollars, he asked for my telephone number so he could let me know on a regular basis how he was getting along. I said, "No, thank you." I didn't know him. Giving him my phone number would have been an expression of compassion without boundaries, *Chesed* , which is a wonderful quality but not appropriate for this occasion. Here I chose to express compassion with boundaries, which is *Tiferet.*

A little further down the map we come to *Netzach,* which means Victory or Endurance and represents a feeling of Firmness. It corresponds to the right hip and leg. This energy can pervert itself into great Egoism if one misuses it by thinking of oneself as "the Victorious one." In that case the energy of *Netzach* needs to be counterbalanced by the energy of the left hip and thigh and leg, which is called *Hod.* Though *Hod* can be translated as Glory, this energy is also Humility. It is God saying, "Don't Glory in your Victory. Don't Glory in your ego."

Next lower on the Tree is the transformer called *Yesod* — corresponding with the penis in men or, in general, the lower abdominal sexual energy. This is also called Foundational energy. This foundational energy can balance Victory and Glory or Victory and Humility.

The tenth *Sefira* is called *Malchut.* I understand it as the Feminine Presence of God within us, the collection of all the energies within us. The word *Malchut* means kingdom. This transformer reminds us to discover/ create the Kingdom of God within ourselves by recognizing the true source of the little "I" within us. While the Crown represents masculine divine energy, *Malchut* represents female energy. We find *Malchut* energy centered at our feet or coccyx. Feminine energy is where the tailbone is or our feet are. (I think that's why many women like shoes so much!)

Every day I pray with people who have various ailments or diseases. I would say seventy percent of my day goes to praying with people in front of the Holy Ark. When I first began my ministry, this was not the case; much of my time went to other rabbinic functions. In the last twenty-five years, my spiritual direction has changed. Our synagogue has hired an assistant rabbi to do a lot of the work I used to do. That allows me to spend more time either meditating with people or doing healing prayer with them. I spend about twelve hours every day doing these spiritual practices.

I also spend quiet time in prayer and meditation before I go to the synagogue, to raise my spiritual vibrations and be sure that my soul is in balance and my soul and body are in balance. When your soul is in balance, when every *Sefira* is in balance with every other *Sefira*, you are correctly aligned spiritually and in a good position to do healing. Just as you have to fill up your car with gasoline if you want to drive, your soul has to receive spiritual energy if you want to do healing. Remember, Kabbalah is about receiving.

There are some wonderful meditations for using the *Sefirot* transformers of energy to heal oneself and others. Here are two very important ones.

HOW TO: Meditation on the Hidden *Sefirot*

Remember, to transmit healing energies effectively to another person, all of your *Sefirot* must be active and in balance. This meditation helps you build the soul muscle to accomplish that.

1. Sit comfortably, keeping your spine straight and your legs, arms, and hands uncrossed. Close your eyes. Focus your attention on your breathing.

2. Bring your awareness to your body. Be aware of the various sensations in and around your body. Then shift your awareness from the physical to the emotional, becoming conscious of the feelings flowing through you.

3. Now focus on your thoughts and try not to think of them from the first-person perspective. Be a witness of them, from the third-person

perspective. Instead of "I think . . ." view them as just thoughts you are seeing.

4. Now move your concentration to focus on the *Sefirot* in sequential order, by focusing on the parts of the body where the corresponding energy centers are.

   A. *Keter – crown*: Slowly lift your attention to the top of your head, to the internal energy center of *Keter*. Perceive a little light, like a ray of light, on the crown of your head. Feel a sense of vibration right there.

   B. *Chochma – right brain*: Perceive a beam of light on the right side of your head and face. At the same time feel vibration in that area, and let that vibration, as well as the light, gently increase in intensity.

   C. *Bina – left brain*: Perceive a beam of light on the left side of your head and face. At the same time feel vibration there, and let it, as well as the light, gently increase in intensity in that area.

   D. Feel the vibrations and sense the light of *Keter, Chochma,* and *Bina* in sequence.

   E. *Chesed – right shoulder*: Visualize a beam of light on your right shoulder. Visualize the beam of light extending down your right arm. At the same time, experience a gentle vibration down your right shoulder and right arm.

   F. *Gevurah/Din – left shoulder*: Visualize a beam of light on your left shoulder and extending down the left arm. At the same time, experience a gentle vibration down your left shoulder and left arm.

   G. *Tiferet – chest*: Visualize a beam of light in the center of your chest, a beam of purple light. Also, feel a sense of vibration gently becoming more and more strong in the solar plexus area.

   H. Feel the vibrations of A–G and visualize the corresponding light in sequence.

   I. *Netzach – right hip*: Visualize a beam of light originating on your right hip and extending down your right thigh and right lower leg. Also, experience a gentle vibration steadily increasing from your right hip down your whole right leg.

J. *Hod – left hip*: Visualize a beam of light originating on your left hip and extending down your left thigh and left lower leg. Also, experience a gentle vibration steadily increasing from your left hip down your whole left leg.

K. *Yesod – lower abdomen*: Focus on your abdominal area, two inches below the belly button. Visualize a beam of light lighting up the area. Also feel a light vibration.

L. Again feel the vibrations of *Keter, Chochma,* and *Bina* and the corresponding light in sequence. Then feel the vibration of *Chesed, Gevurah/Din, Tiferet,* and the corresponding light in sequence. Then feel the vibration of *Netzach, Hod,* and *Yesod* and the corresponding light in sequence.

M. *Malchut – coccyx*: Finally, move your awareness from the base of the abdomen to the base of the spine, the coccyx, by feeling a slight pressure there and visualizing light in that area. Then feel the light move through both legs and into your feet.

N. Again, allow yourself to perceive light and vibrations in each *Sefira,* corresponding to the different parts of the body, corresponding to the *Sefirot* of the Soul.

5. Feel all your *Sefirot* at once now. Feel your soul vibrating. You are now exercising your soul. When you do this, you are putting yourself in a position to bring healing to another person with the spiritual vibrations of your soul, because all your *Sefirot* are in spiritual balance. This is one way to activate your *Sefirot* — to increase the vibrational energy of your soul with which to heal.

Here is an alternative method to increase the vibrational energy of your soul and create soul balance. Rabbi Yaakov taught me this meditation, based on *Sefer Yetzirah* Ch. 1, *Mishna* 9. It recognizes that the breath of the living God can be drawn into the individual through his or her crown, or *Keter*. Here we relate *Ru'ach elohim hayim* to God's Hebrew name *Yah* (*Sefer Yetzirah* Ch, 1, *Mishna* 9 maintains that the first name of God is *Yah*). *Ru'ach* means breath, as God's breath. *Elohim* means God, as Judge; *Hayim* means life, as God is life.

In this meditation, we identify our breath with God's breath. By doing so, we activate and energize and balance the Soul of our body.

HOW TO: **Fill Yourself Up with the Breath of the Living God,
Activating Your *Sefirot***

1. Recognize and be aware that the breath of the Living God is every-where. Indeed, God is as close to you as the air in your lungs and all around you. God is Breath.

2. Sit in a comfortable place, in a comfortable chair, with your back upright. If possible, loosen your belt. As you sit, imagine that attached to your feet and going through the floor of the room are energy legs and energy feet, touching the earth. You and your soul are now an intermediary between God's celestial energy and God's earthly energy.

3. Mentally speak the word *Ru'ach,* and then inhale gently through your nostrils. As you inhale, visualize God's celestial breath/energy/light coming through *Keter,* the crown of your head, filling your head, being drawn down into your heart, and filling your heart.

4. As you feel the breath of God in your heart area, hold your breath to the count of three and mentally say *Elohim* while you do so. At the same time, visualize your heart filled with the breath of God/light/energy.

5. Exhale gently through your nostrils. As you do so, mentally say the word *Hayim* and visualize God's breath leaving your heart, going through your abdomen, through your legs, through your feet, then on through your energy legs and energy feet (imaginary legs and imaginary feet) into the earth.

6. Feel that God's energy has been drawn down throughout your whole body, through the crown of your head, through your heart, through your abdomen, through your legs, into the earth. At the same time, know that the *Sefirot* of your soul have been activated, transforming God's breath/energy into *Sefirotic* energy from your head to your toes.

7. Repeat steps 3–6 four more times, so that you have done them each five times altogether.

8. Now, breathe in gently through your nostrils and, as you do so, mentally say *Ru'ach* and visualize or feel God's earth energy going *up* through your energy feet, energy legs, real feet, real legs, into your heart. Hold your breath for about three seconds and see your heart filled with light/energy/breath as you say mentally the word *Elohim*.

9. As you gently exhale through your nostrils, visualize God's breath/ energy/light moving up from your heart into your head, and then moving out of your head upward through *Keter*. As it moves up from your heart, through your head, through the crown of your head, see God's energy/light separate as a light fountain — one half of the light fountain goes to the left, the other to the right.

10. Repeat steps 8–9 four more times so that you have a total of five times for each of them.

11. Repeat steps 3–9 five times.

We exercise our soul fifteen times in this meditation, because the Hebrew word *Yah*, which *Sefer Yetzirah* calls God's first name, has the numerical equivalence of 15. (*Yod* has the numerical value of 10. *Hey* has the numerical value of 5.) The ancient *Sefer Yetzirah* also correlates God's name *Yah* with another of God's Hebrew names, *Ru'ach elohim hayim*. Our mystic texts have a plethora of Hebrew holy names for God. Each has its own unique meaning. This meditation brings Balance to you and the energy of your *Sefirot*, and also brings Balance between God's celestial energy and God's earthly energy within you.

You may do either or both of these two meditation exercises above to strengthen the *Sefirot* of your soul. Perhaps you would do one on Monday and Wednesday and the other on Tuesday and Thursday. It's good to know and master many kinds of spiritual therapies and modalities so you can become an expert. More important than just knowing these modalities is practicing, practicing, and practicing them so you own them.

There are many modalities of Balance. In our context, Balance means that all the *Sefirot* within you are in balance — especially that their energies are in balance vis-à-vis the energy of God. You can't give balance to another if you don't have it yourself. That's why it's so important to do these spiritual exercises at home daily.

It's also important to develop a relationship with God, and thank God daily for what you have. You need to have a balanced relationship with God, and to be a good person. Share what you have with others, whether friends or strangers.

Now I would like to share another modality with you — similar, but different from the ones above. This one places *YHVH* יהוה, the Face of God, on each of our *Sefirot*. It is called a *Merkavah,* a Chariot of God meditation. Placing this Manifestation of God on the energy centers of our body, and identifying it with them, is a most powerful way to become God-filled.

Rabbi Dan Dresher and Rabbi Dr. Yaakov Dresher both shared this powerful meditation with me. It derives from Rabbi Chaim Vital's sixteenth-century sacred text, *Ru'ach HaKodesh,* in which Rabbi Vital shares what he learned from the greatest Kabbalistic teacher of all, Rabbi Isaac Luria.

I do this meditation more often than any other, almost every morning. It not only reminds me that God is within me from head to toe, it activates and balances the *Sefirotic* energies of my body and soul and binds me ever so strongly with the energies of God. Every time I do healing prayer with someone, I recollect this meditation from earlier in the morning; this recollection greatly helps me be a vessel for the Divine . . . a chariot for the Presence of God.

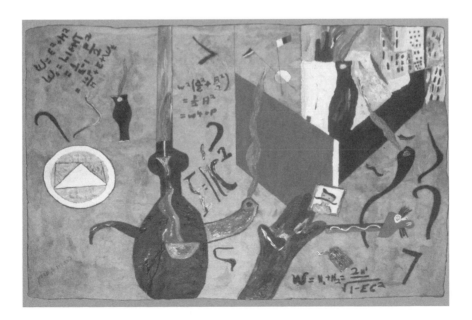

HOW TO: A *Merkavah* Meditation, Making You a Chariot of God by Identifying the Energies of *YHVH* with the Ten *Sefirot*

This meditation not only fills us with the Presence of God, it also has the effect of creating balance within the flow of divine energy of God. It is based on a principle from the *Zohar* that our actions below have a direct effect on the celestial world. We strengthen enormously our connection with God in this meditation. Refer to the Chariot of God illustration above on page 121.

1. *Keter* First visualize sets of *YHVH* יהוה in translucent gold color, circling your head counterclockwise like a halo. Recite Psalm 16:8, "I place *YHVH* before me always." Or, preferably, say it in Hebrew: *Shiviti YHVH l'negdi tamid.* I believe that, effective as it is in English, it is even more effective in Hebrew, because when you pronounce the Hebrew words, you also activate the vibrational powers of the Hebrew letters.

2. *Chochma*
   A. Visualize *YHVH* יהוה in white letters about five inches in front of your right forehead.
   B. Say *I place YHVH before me always* or, preferably, *Shiviti YHVH l'negdi tamid.*
   C. Breathe in gently through your nostrils and visualize the image of *YHVH* יהוה in white characters moving toward your right forehead and affixing itself to it.
   D. Breathe out gently through your nostrils and see *YHVH* יהוה in white characters firmly established on your right forehead.

3. *Bina*
   A. Visualize *YHVH* יהוה in green letters about five inches in front of your left forehead.
   B. Say *I place YHVH before me always* or, preferably, *Shiviti YHVH l'negdi tamid.*
   C. Breathe in through your nostrils and visualize the green *YHVH* יהוה moving toward your left forehead and affixing itself to it.
   D. Breathe out through your nostrils and see the green *YHVH* יהוה firmly established on your left forehead.

4. *Chesed*
   A. Visualize *YHVH* יהוה in light blue letters about five inches in front of your right shoulder.
   B. Say *I place YHVH before me always* or, preferably, *Shiviti YHVH l'negdi tamid.*
   C. Breathe in through your nostrils and visualize the light blue *YHVH* יהוה moving toward your right shoulder and affixing itself to it.
   D. Breathe out through your nostrils and visualize many sets of *YHVH* יהוה in light blue characters moving down your right arm.

5. *Gevurah/Din*
   A. Visualize *YHVH* יהוה in deep red letters about five inches in front of your left shoulder.
   B. Say *I place YHVH before me always* or, preferably, *Shiviti YHVH l'negdi tamid.*
   C. Breathe in through your nostrils and visualize the deep red *YHVH* יהוה moving toward your left shoulder and affixing itself to it.
   D. Breathe out through your nostrils and visualize many sets of *YHVH* יהוה in deep red characters moving down your left arm.

6. *Tiferet*
   A. Visualize *YHVH* יהוה in purple letters about five inches in front of your solar plexus.
   B. Say *I place YHVH before me always* or, preferably, *Shiviti YHVH l'negdi tamid.*
   C. Breathe in through your nostrils and visualize the purple *YHVH* יהוה moving onto your solar plexus.
   D. Breathe out through your nostrils and visualize many sets of *YHVH* יהוה in purple characters firmly affixed to your solar plexus.

7. *Netzach*
   A. Visualize *YHVH* יהוה in dark pink letters about five inches in front of your right hip.
   B. Say *I place YHVH before me always* or, preferably, *Shiviti YHVH l'negdi tamid.*
   C. Breathe in through your nostrils and visualize the dark pink

YHVH יהוה moving toward your right hip and affixing itself to it.

D. Breathe out through your nostrils and visualize many sets of *YHVH* יהוה in dark pink characters moving down your right hip, down your right leg, to your ankle.

8. *Hod*

A. Visualize *YHVH* יהוה in light pink letters about five inches in front of your left hip.

B. Say *I place YHVH before me always* or, preferably, *Shiviti YHVH l'negdi tamid.*

C. Breathe in through your nostrils and visualize the light pink *YHVH* יהוה moving toward your left hip and affixing itself to it.

D. As you breathe out through your nostrils, visualize many sets of *YHVH* יהוה in light pink characters moving down your left hip, down your left leg, to your ankle.

9. *Yesod*

A. Visualize *YHVH* יהוה in orange letters about three inches in front of your lower abdomen.

B. Say *I place YHVH before me always* or, preferably, *Shiviti YHVH l'negdi tamid.*

C. Breathe in through your nostrils and visualize the orange *YHVH* יהוה moving toward your lower abdomen and affixing itself to it.

D. Breathe out through your nostrils and visualize *YHVH* יהוה in orange characters directly affixed on your lower abdomen.

10. *Malchut*

A. Visualize *YHVH* יהוה in navy blue letters on each foot.

B. Say *I place YHVH before me always* or, preferably, *Shiviti YHVH l'negdi tamid.*

C. Breathe in through your nostrils and visualize the navy blue *YHVH* יהוה on your feet.

D. Breathe out through your nostrils and visualize again *YHVH* יהוה in navy blue characters directly on each foot.

Know that you and *Hashem* are completely in sync. Know also that all your *Sefirot* are in balance. Finally, know that, just as you've inspired your *Sefirot* to be in balance with one another, you have inspired balance in what is now manifesting in the Mind of God. "As above, so below; as below, so above."

The Third Eye or *Da'at* Consciousness

One afternoon some years ago, it snowed quite heavily in Washington, D.C. I had been visiting with Rabbi Yaakov for several days and was scheduled to leave. Unfortunately, no flights were leaving Reagan National Airport. Rabbi Yaakov kindly offered to let me stay another day or two.

We sat relaxed in the living room, in front of the fireplace. I asked him a question that had been bothering me, "Rabbi, do we Jews believe in the Third Eye? How can we achieve the vision and wisdom that some people speak of in that way? And can you teach me how to do it?"

Before I could utter my next question, Rabbi Yaakov smiled and said, "Slow down, Douglas. We can achieve similar results, but we don't call it the Third Eye. We call it *Da'at* consciousness." Then he opened his *Sefer Yetzirah* and read to me from Ch.1, *Mishna* 4:

> Ten *Sefirot* of nothingness
> Ten and not nine
> Ten and not eleven
> Understand with wisdom
> Be wise with understanding
> Examine with them
> And probe them. . . .

"To understand how we can achieve what you call the Third Eye, Douglas," he continued, "and what we call *Da'at* consciousness, we need to understand the difference between *Chochma* and *Bina*."

He then explained to me again that within the human body, the *Sefirotic* energies polarize in columns of right and left, and these energies are always vibrating. When we balance these energies through meditative practices and prayer, we achieve physical health. The *Mishna* from *Sefer Yetzirah* that he read specifically mentions two of the *Sefirot: Chochma,* Wisdom, and *Bina,* Understanding.

On the level of *Chochma,* past, present, and future have not yet been separated. This Wisdom corresponds to our right brain functioning. It is Spirit, superior to intellect, and masculine. We call it *Abba,* or Father. Its mode of communication is nonverbal. We often speak of it as the unconscious part of the human mind.

Bina, in contrast, is a level lower and functions as what we normally speak of as the conscious part of the human mind. At this level we understand ideas separately, whereas *Chochma*/Wisdom is a mode of undifferentiated Mind. *Bina*/Understanding is the aspect of mind where division exists, where things are defined and experienced as separate objects. *Bina* is feminine and we call it *Imma* or Mother. *Bina*/Understanding is seen as the rational mind. *Chochma*/Wisdom is seen as the intuitive mind.

Chochma and *Bina* are not only two modes of the human mind, but more primarily are two modes of the mind of God. Kabbalah teaches that *Chochma* and *Bina* are always together. They never part. A profound Kabbalistic secret used in healing is that *Da'at,* or Knowledge, though not a *Sefira* in itself, is the place where *Chochma* and *Bina* unite. In the realm of *Da'at,* right and left brain come together.

Holographically, even though *Chochma* is an independent *Sefira,* some aspects of it can be caught within *Bina. Da'at,* or Knowledge, as the lower manifestation of *Keter,* is what captures the united power of *Chochma* and *Bina.* Though *Chochma* and *Bina* are not the same, we can inspire *Chochma* and *Bina* to work together in a harmony that allows *Bina* to reveal *Chochma* and allows *Chochma* to reveal *Bina* in a dynamic back-and-forth consciousness. This comes about through the power of "Knowledge" that is a union of *Chochma* and *Bina.*

Through a specific meditative experience, through altered states of consciousness that move between *Chochma* consciousness and *Bina* consciousness, we receive *Da'at* or the Third Eye wisdom. The life-energy forces of *Chochma* and *Bina* operating in *Da'at* consciousness allow us to understand our world from a unique perspective of great spiritual health.

HOW TO: **Meditation on the Third Eye**

1. Go to your *mi'at meekdash.* Sit comfortably in loose clothing with your belt unbuckled.

2. Close your eyes and first focus above your right eyebrow on your right-brain, *Chochma*-level of consciousness.

3. Breathe in gently and deeply through your nostrils.

4. As you breathe out, make the sound *mmmmmmmm.* Feel your whole body from head to toe vibrate.

5. Now focus above your left eyebrow. Know that you are focusing on your left brain, your *Bina* level of consciousness.

6. Breathe in gently and deeply through your nostrils.

7. As you breathe out, make the sound *shhhhhh,* the sound of *shin.*

8. Do this oscillating back and forth from *Chochma* consciousness to *Bina* consciousness, at least twenty-six times, if not more.

9. Focus now on the middle, between both eyebrows, between *Chochma* and *Bina.* Know that through the oscillation of your consciousness here from one to the other, *Chochma* is revealed in *Bina* and *Bina* is revealed in *Chochma.* Wisdom is revealed in Understanding and Understanding is revealed within Wisdom.

10. Continue to focus on the middle. Notice that both your eyes are now focused on the Third Eye. They are not to move. This middle place, or *Da'at,* which unites *Chochma* and *Bina,* is drawing strength into itself from the energy of *Keter.* This is your Third Eye. The more you focus on it, the more it becomes alive.

11. As you continue to focus on *Da'at,* your gaze will become even more fixed. Through *Da'at,* you will see things for the first time that you never saw before. You are being introduced to a new form of sight. Not the sight of ordinary vision, it is the sight of the *mind.* You will see thoughts running before you and you will become witness to those thoughts.

―――――――――――

Normally you identify with your thoughts. If there is anger, you become angry. If there is joy, you become joyful. Normally, you become one with the thought to the extent that you become the thought, that you identify with it. There is then no gap between you and the thought. But when you focus on *Da'at,* you become a witness. You see your thoughts moving like cars on a highway — this is one of the amazing effects of the life energies of *Chochma* and *Bina* within us.

"Energy flows where attention goes," Rabbi Yaakov said numerous times. "Understand with Wisdom. Be wise with Understanding. Energy flows where attention goes." As you become a witness centered in the Third Eye of *Da'at,* healing happens.

Let's say, for example, you are sick with the flu. Your legs hurt, your head aches. When you are in the Third Eye, however, you are a witness to your flu. You are not identifying with it. Be such a witness. Be an observer. Embrace healing.

In the Third Eye, when *Chochma* and *Bina* are united each in one another, imagination and actualization are not two things. Imagination and actualization are one. This is because we find *Hashem* in the Third Eye. Therefore, just imagining that God's healing light is showering you from the top of your head to the bottom of your feet allows God's light to do this. And you and God are one in healing.

NOTE

1. A long scroll with the entire text of the Five Books of Moses hand-written in the original Hebrew, rolled around two beautifully designed wooden spools.

9

Healing Properties of
the Hebrew Calendar

I OFTEN do the *Shiviti* meditation in the morning: *Shiviti YHVH l'negdi tamid, I place YHVH before me always.* This healing prayer creates balance within my *Sefirot*, which allows me to do healing blessings during the day. I also sometimes do the *Shiviti* meditation with a person who is receiving healing.

Each person's soul is different and is at a different *madreyga,* or level. I believe everyone has a unique spiritual DNA in the souls of their cells, just as they have a unique chemical DNA in their cellular structure. Because of this, no one healing meditation fits all. Some people respond to one spiritual exercise and readily embrace it, while others embrace a different one with greater joy and greater faith. It's as if their cellular structure is magnetically attracted to a certain exercise.

Over the years, many people I've prayed with have loved doing the *Shiviti* prayer. We sit in front of the Holy Ark and visualize together the *YHVH* energies embracing their corresponding *Sefirot*. It is powerful. When I do it alone in the morning, it is an equally powerful method of meeting and embracing God.

The *Shiviti YHVH* meditation inspires us to feel God's Presence very strongly. I began noticing, though, about five years ago, that our results of praying with it were uneven. There were times when we had great results, with the diminution of tumors, and other times when the tumors did not shrink at all. I felt that difference was in part due to the spiritual DNA of the person I was praying for. So in cases where it wasn't working, we abandoned this *Shiviti* modality and changed to an entirely new spiritual protocol. My prayer partner frequently improved in health with the new prayer arrangement.

I intuitively felt, though, that the *Shiviti* prayer is so powerful that it should have worked, and that maybe I wasn't doing it in the best possible way. I didn't know what "best possible way" meant, but I had a gut feeling that at times I wasn't doing it to its maximum capacity.

I felt this especially strongly about three years ago when praying with a young woman named Barbara who suffered from tumors in the lower left part of her abdomen. When she first came to me, Barbara continued with her medical protocol as I introduced her to different healing meditations. We did Jeremiah's *Refa'einu* prayer (which we discuss in Chapter 14 as Jeremiah's healing prayer) in several variations. Before we did that, though, we always sat together in front of the Ark and did the *Shiviti* meditation together. Both of us felt connected to God, which allowed us to feel very receptive to Jeremiah's prayer.

In the first year of combining this spiritual protocol with her medical regimen, she was feeling great. Even though her tumors did not diminish in size, she was living a life without symptoms. She had no pain, she had no more nausea, and she once again played golf. Her mental outlook was excellent. The pictures showed tumors, but she herself was living an asymptomatic life. Her physicians were surprised, but told her to continue whatever she was doing.

Barbara realized that with God activated within her, she could embrace the world with great joy . . . until her tumors began to grow again. I was puzzled, because I strongly felt we were doing the right thing. I had every confidence that not only would she feel better, but that she would be better. I instinctively knew that the tumors would diminish in size. Things appeared to have been going great, but the tumors began to get larger again — Why would that be? She embraced *Hashem*. She identified *Hashem*, God's Face of *YHVH*, with every *Sefira* on her body.

I shared all this with Rabbi Yaakov, as I believed it to be very unusual. I also shared with him that, when I did the *Shiviti* prayer with Barbara, the divine flow within me was uneven. I did not feel the same inner strength of divine flow every month. Some months I felt more connected to God while doing this prayer than during other months, when I felt less connected to God. I said, "I know it sounds strange, it sounds crazy, but it's as if I feel a different divine energy flow when the Jewish month changes." And yet, I didn't want to abandon the *Shiviti* prayer. There was something within me that kept insisting that I continue to embrace the *Shiviti* meditation.

Rabbi Yaakov responded, "You are right. It's all about the month. You intuited correctly."

"I don't understand."

"Are you familiar with Rabbi Tzvi Elimelech Shapira's *Bnei Yissa'char?*"

I told him I had heard of Rabbi Shapira, also known as the Dynover Reb (1783–1841), and that I knew that he was best known for his work, the *Bnei Yissa'char.* When we first began our synagogue, one of our members, Corinne Shapira, often told me of her illustrious rabbinic family. She was very proud of the Dynover Reb and his Kabbalistic masterpiece *Bnei Yissa'char,* which is a commentary on the Torah and Festivals from a Kabbalistic perspective.

Rabbi Yaakov shared with me that the Dynover Reb taught that God's energy manifests itself in time, just as it is realized in space, and that we need to feel the Divine Pulse during every moment of time. Furthermore, the Dynover Reb taught that every month corresponds to a different permutation of the Divine Name *YHVH.*

Technically, the Jewish calendar is based on the cycles of the moon, with modifications that are based on the solar cycle. Because of differences in the solar and lunar calendars, there is no exact correlation between the Jewish calendar and the Gregorian calendar that most countries follow. Some years Chanukah (the 25th day of the Jewish month *Kislev*) coincides with Christmas (the 25th day of December in the Gregorian calendar). Another year, it may coincide with Thanksgiving (and gets nicknamed Thanksgivukkah). The Jewish calendar also adds an extra month, a "leap" month, as needed to stay in sync with the solar cycle, much as the Gregorian calendar adds a leap day every four years.

However, at its heart, it is a spiritual calendar. I say this because each month of the Jewish year is reflected by a different spelling of the *Tetragrammaton.* There are twelve permutations of the *Tetragrammaton,* and each spelling connects us to the inner purpose of each month of the year. The mysticism of this brings down God's transcendental light into each life when we say the *Birkat HaChodesh,* Blessing of the Month, and *Birkat HaLevanah,* Blessing of the Moon, when we focus on one of these twelve permutations. Thus it is a spiritual calendar that governs the workings of our months.

The Dynover Reb teaches that in every month of the lunar calendar, *YHVH,* the holy letters of God's face and their corresponding energies manifest in a different permutation. In other words, in each month, a different combination of the letters of God's name is manifest — twelve months, twelve combinations of God's name. The Dynover Reb looks into the Hebrew word for month, *chodesh,* and shows that it derives from the Hebrew word *chadash,* which means new, implying a different energy in every month. That is, the change in the holy letters or energies of God's name in each month brings into existence a new aspect of God's being or a different smile to God's face.

Rabbi Yaakov explained in this way why I felt the Divine Energies varied every month with the *Shiviti* prayer. It was because God's energies are not equally or optimally accessible when we call upon God by visualizing the *YHVH* in the same sequence every month. He said that even though Barbara and I had been praying with the right *kavvanah* — with belief, with the Greater Mind, and with the right faith — we did not receive a positive response because we did not use the exact Name of *Hashem* for that specific month.

Psalm 91 teaches: "Because he is devoted to Me, I will deliver him; I will keep him safe because he knows My Name. When he calls on Me, I will answer him" (Psalm 91:14–15). The Dynover Reb teaches, by referring to this Psalm, that if we call upon God by the appropriate Name, the appropriate permutation of *YHVH,* our prayers will be heard and answered.

We need to realize always that when we internalize the Hebrew letters that make up God's name, we are not internalizing *letters* per se, but *energies.* To call upon God accurately, we need to call upon the sequence of energies that make up how God is manifesting for that particular month — in the most accurate way possible.

Hashem manifests one way at Rosh Hashanah and another at Passover. *Hashem* manifests one way during the month of *Iyar* and differently in *Sivan*, and still differently in *Kislev* and *Tevet*. If we want the healing energy of *Hashem* to flow within us, we need to attune to the Divine Presence as it manifests that month. That's why the Torah maintains "And I prayed to God *at that time*" (Deut. 3:23).

What does "at that time" mean? The Dynover Reb teaches that Moses prayed to God "at that time" by calling upon God with the specific permutation of the Ineffable Name for that month, the specific permutation at that time.

Now, when I come across the Ineffable Name, *YHVH*, in different prayers, the prayer of Jeremiah or any other healing prayer that uses the *YHVH*, I first recite the prayer as it is in the text, and then I recite the prayer visualizing the permutation that is specific to that month. For example, the *Refa'einu* prayer reads:

> *Refa'einu Adonai 1 v'neirafeh hoshi'einu v'nivashe'ah ki t'hilateinu atah v'ha'aleh refuah shleimah l'chol makoteinu ki el melech rofeh v'ne'eman v'rachaman atah. Baruch atah Adonai rofeh cholim.*

> *Heal us, Lord, and we shall be healed. Save us and we shall be saved, for You are our praise. Bring complete recovery for all our ailments, for You, God, King, are a faithful and compassionate Healer. Blessed are You, Lord, YHVH, Healer of the sick.*

The Dynover Reb not only describes the accessible divine energies of the *YHVH* in each month, he also identifies the letter of the *alef bet* (alphabet) with which that month was created. The permutations he provides appear in the table below. I first say the prayer as it is originally written, and then — depending what month it is during which I am praying — I say it again with the appropriate permutation from the table below.

For example, if it is the month of *Iyar*, I say יההו; if it is the month of *Sivan*, I say יוהה.

Hebrew letter with which month created	YHVH Permutation	Jewish Month	Length— number of days	English Equivalent
ה	יהוה	Nissan	30	March - April
ו	יההו	Iyar	29	April - May
ז	יוהה	Sivan	30	May - June
ח	הוהי	Tammuz	29	June - July
פ	הויה	Av	30	July - August
ף	ההוי	Elul	29	August - Sept.
ל	והיה	Tishri	30	Sept. – Oct.
נ	וההי	Cheshvan	29 or 30	Oct. – Nov.
ם	ויהה	Kislev	30 or 29	Nov. – Dec.
ץ	היהו	Tevet	29	Dec. – Jan.
צ	היוה	Shevat	30	Jan. – Feb.
ק	ההיו	Adar	29 or 30	Feb. – March

NOTE

1. The Hebrew word *Adonai* corresponds to one of the twelve sequences of *YHVH*. So, if I am saying this prayer in the month of *Nissan*, I visualize *YHVH* יהוה. If I am saying the prayer in the month of *Iyar*, I first recite the prayer as written, and then repeat the prayer, this time visualizing *YHHV* יההו when I say the word *Adonai* and so on.

10

The Power of Hands

SINCE I was a little boy, I have been aware of my hands. I was born in 1945 with an extended strawberry birthmark that fully covered my left hand and arm. The attending physician told my parents that the birthmark on my hand could be eradicated by recently developed radiation technology. My parents consented when I was thirty days old.

Through a series of errors, the radiation used in those techniques burned my left hand. I had numerous hand surgeries in my formative years to correct the radiation burns. By high school, other than the scarring and the birthmark which did not disappear, my left hand was as good as new and I played baseball, violin, and hockey. But I was always conscious and aware of my "red hand." I knew my hands were different than other people's.

My mother always warned me about keeping my hand out of the sun when I was little. She wanted my hand covered, for fear I might get cancer. When I was older, I hid my left hand in my pocket, especially when meeting girls for the first time.

It never occurred to me before I was ordained that, unlike rabbis who use their mouths to preach, I would use my hands to teach and preach — because my first pulpit was a deaf congregation. Because of the needs of my community, I had to interpret Hebrew prayers and Biblical texts in American Sign Language, the language of hands. At that time, in 1972, there were no rabbis serving the Jewish deaf community. I thought this would be a wonderful opportunity not only to serve a minority within Judaism, but also a great privilege to serve God by ministering to many of His people who had not yet been taught Torah.

When I assumed my pulpit more than forty years ago and began communicating all my lectures, lessons, and sermons in sign language, it felt as
if I were healing through my hands. My hands, which were once hidden,
became prominent. They conveyed the word of God. They brought spiritual
healing to a community that had been spiritually fractured and without an
ordained rabbi. Little did I know that my hands eventually would become
instruments of God's healing for people of all faiths.

Only in later years did I learn that fingers are closely related to the power of
speech. The Kabbalah teaches that the concealed becomes revealed through
one's hands: The ten fingers represent the ten energies or *Sefirot* through
which God can be revealed.

This learning began in earnest when I met Rabbi Dan Dresher and he
taught me the healing prayer of Moses. I used that prayer so often that
it became an essential part of my rabbinate; because of it, my ministry
truly became a healing ministry. Years later, the younger Rabbi Dr. Yaakov
Dresher continued to mentor me in Kabbalistic techniques of healing
prayer. Both men taught me that a person's hands can bring God's blessings
into this world. When we literally raise our hands to God, we recognize
that there is a God and we convey our own recognition of God to others.

Our synagogue Shabbat services are extremely lively, filled with the spirit
of humanity and God. People can't help but feel the spirit of the *Shechina*
as we clap to the beat of the sacred tunes being sung and signed by the
congregation. Over the last ten years, the demographics of our congregation have changed to include many hearing people in addition to our deaf
members. Voices and hands are both raised in praise to God. Often people
tell me, "The services feel so Evangelical or Baptist."

Perhaps they do. But our clapping and dancing and singing and signing actually have deep Kabbalistic roots. Rabbi Nachman of Breslov, the
great Kabbalistic teacher, wrote extensively about the spiritual importance
of hands in healing. "When two hands clap against one another, the five
fingers of the right hand meet the five fingers of the left hand — that is
5×5. In the reverse meeting, when the left hand meets the right, that is
also 5×5. And 2×25 in *gematria* equals 50." Rabbi Nachman goes on
to say that this 50 parallels the fiftieth gate which was revealed by God to

bring the greatest healing. He teaches that, when we clap our hands during our prayers, we inspire the power of salvation and hasten our redemption. There is healing in our hands.

Kabbalistic tradition teaches that every being — even trees and plants with healing properties — has spirit guides. In an ancient Hebrew commentary on our Torah, *Bereshit Rabba* 10:6, we learn there is nothing below which does not have an angel on high that strikes it and strokes it and tells it to grow.

The power of the angels to communicate life energy is referred to in Kabbalistic literature as the power of the hands. Just as the angels bless with their hands, we humans bless with our hands. Just as angels contain life force within them, we contain life force within our hands. Psalm 145:16 teaches, "You open Your hands and satiate all living beings, according to Your will." Since we are created in God's image and with God's soul, we too can open our hands and bring healing to human beings. I have learned and seen that our hands, when raised to God, can bring healing and blessing into the world. The more people raise their hands in prayer, and the more we bless one another with our hands, the more healing is bestowed on Earth.

There will come a day that people will be free to use their hands for prayer and blessing instead of only for physical work in the toil of factory and field. We one day will use our hands, all of us, to attain spirituality. Not only surgeons will use their hands for healing, ordinary people like you and me will pray for one another and bless one another so that healing will take place. Truly, each human being, regardless of religion or race, has hands that heal.

As I've said before, every Hebrew letter has a numerical value, and Kabbalists find mystical meanings in the numerical value of Hebrew words — a practice called *gematria*. Let's look at some more examples of it.

In the Five Books of Moses, the Hebrew root of the word for healing — *Refuah, RFA* — appears fourteen times. The numerical value of the word for hand is 14. The mystical interpretation of this occurrence is that there is a unique relationship between healing and hands.

Rabbi Nachman of Breslov celebrates the importance of hands in healing in a prayer I learned from Rabbi Yaakov. Before I do healing work on anyone, I always pray this prayer:

> Our God and God of our fathers, bless me and bless my hands, that I might become a pure instrument of your healing light, so that your healing/light energy flows through me, and through my hands, bringing complete healing to the person I am praying for.

Remember — if you don't have a powerful relationship with God, you cannot be a powerful healer. A powerful relationship with God includes regular talking and praying and meditating with God every morning. It also means being kind and more kind to people on a regular basis. *It won't work any other way.* Even if your car is a Jaguar, you need gasoline to make it work. Even if you are an intuitive person, a natural in healing, you need to fill yourself up every day with the fuel of being in love with God and in love with people.

Jewish healing tradition teaches that when one person prays or blesses another person, this is a level of "Seeing God." In the book of Hosea (12:11) we read, "Through the hands of the prophets I cause an image to be seen." Consider that as you read these next several paragraphs.

Rabbi Dan Dresher taught me that when I pray for healing I should stretch forth my arms to the heavens, with my palms facing upwards, and imagine two columns of bright light coming down from the heavens into the palms of my hands. He taught me to concentrate with *kavvanah* on the two columns of light, feeling the warmth of the light in the palms of my hands. And as I feel the warm light, I should recognize and know that I am making contact with the Divine Presence.

Rabbi Yaakov later alerted me to a wonderful insight. He asked me to hold my hands facing each other in front of me at chest level, about fifteen inches apart. He asked me to keep my fingers together as my palms faced each other. He then asked me to move my hands closer and farther apart, like playing an accordion. He asked me to do this very slowly, feeling the energy of the *Sefirot* between my palms and fingers. When I brought my hands closer together, I felt the energy very strongly. As I moved them farther apart, I felt a decrease in the strength of the energy.

Rabbi Yaakov then asked me to look at the diagram of the *Sefirot* and transfer the *Sefirot* from the right column to the fingers of my right hand and the *Sefirot* of the left column to the fingers of my left hand. The right hand with its fingers represents the masculine *Sefirot* and the left hand with its fingers represents the feminine *Sefirot*. He said then to identify each of my ten fingers with the respective *Sefira*. I did.

Then, as I moved my hands back and forth, the energy field between my hands was much stronger than in our first exercise. I was aware of the different *Sefirot* in my hands. I saw again that they could channel God's light and God's energy.

Since all beings are made up of the Hebrew letters and the *Sefirot*, the energy of the letters flows constantly within us and is regularly adjusted or transformed by our inner *Sefirot*. Notice the letters in the diagram on page 149. Their placement helps us see how we, and all beings, are made up spiritually of the energies of the Hebrew letters and the transformers of these energies called *Sefirot*. The flow of energy occurs through different channels or *tzinorot*.

When these channels are open and allow for free-flowing circulation of God's *Ru'ach* or energy, God's light is in complete balance within us. We are in harmony within ourselves and with God. We are receiving God's light and the light flows unhindered through us. When there is free flow, when the channels are not blocked, when the *Ru'ach* flows freely, unhindered within us, we are healthy. We are in a state of equilibrium.

Praying for healing with members of my community involves using my hands to transfer God's healing to the person I'm with. Sometimes I feel that changing my own inner flow of energy from a state of equilibrium to a state of tension will help me channel God's healing light or healing energy more powerfully.

> Ten *Sefirot* of Nothingness
> In the number of ten fingers
> Five opposite five
> With a singular covenant
> Precisely in the middle . . .
> —*Sefer Yetzirah,* Chapter 1, *Mishna* 3

This *Mishna* completely changes the traditional way of viewing the *Sefirot*. Normally we see the flow of divine energy in three columns, as in the Tree of Life diagram. In this familiar pattern the flow is a free, unhindered balance of energy. The *Sefirot* are in a state of equilibrium, and the individual is experiencing good health. This is what we want the recipient of our healing to look like.

However, if we want to deliver God's healing to another person, we need to bring the energies of the *Sefirot* into two columns. Doing this creates a state of tension in the energy within us; and we become a unique instrument that can channel God's healing energy to another person.

In people who are ill, their channels for the free flow of God's energy, or *Ru'ach,* are blocked. Rabbi Yaakov showed me how, using the *Mishna* above, I could unblock the flow of the sick person's energy by changing into such an instrument. Here is how to arrange the divine energies into the two columns for healing.

Each column is represented by five fingers. We are to see the masculine *Sefirot* in the five digits of the right hand. These include the three *Sefirot* on the right column of the Tree of Life diagram, and the upper two *Sefirot* of the middle column. We see the feminine *Sefirot* in the fingers and thumb of the left hand. These include the three *Sefirot* in the left column of the Tree of Life diagram, and the two lower *Sefirot* in the middle column of the diagram.

Rabbi Yaakov showed me the Biblical text of Isaiah which speaks of how God created the world with His hands, "My left hand has founded the Earth and my right hand has spread out the heavens" (Isaiah 48:13). Since we are created in God's image, we too can create with our hands, using our God-given energies.

I learned this Kabbalistic secret of healing — creating a model of two columns of *Sefirotic* energy — several years after writing my first book. I have experienced wonderful results using this technique.

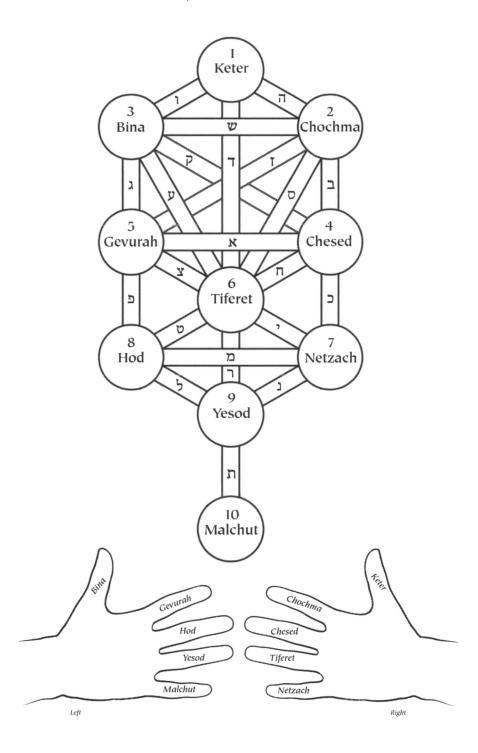

HOW TO: Meditation to Feel Divine Energy

1. Sit in a comfortable chair in a comfortable place, with your back upright. If possible, loosen your pants or unbuckle your belt.

2. Recognize and be aware that the breath of the Living God is everywhere, that God is as close to you as the air you breathe. God is Breath. Inhale and exhale slowly through your nostrils, breathing God's *Ru'ach* within yourself.

3. Place your hands at chest level, about fifteen inches apart, with your fingers closed and your palms facing each other. Move your hands back and forth from fifteen inches to four inches. Feel the energy between them become more intense as your hands are closer together and less intense as they are further apart.

4. To increase your awareness of the divine energy within you, press the thumb of your right hand into the center of your left palm. Do this for three seconds. Then press the thumb of your left hand into the center of your right palm. Do this for three seconds.

5. You are now ready to channel and direct divine energy to the person you are praying with for healing.

HOW TO: Increase the Voltage of Divine Energy

1–2. Repeat steps 1 and 2 above.

3. Put your hands in front of you fifteen inches apart and identify the five masculine *Sefirot* with the five digits of your right hand and the five feminine *Sefirot* with the five digits of your left hand (see page 149). As you imagine the *Sefirot* corresponding to the fingers and thumb of each hand, you are polarizing these *Sefirot* and creating strong spiritual tension. This tension is the divine energy within you.

4. To increase your awareness of this energy within you, press the thumb of your right hand into the center of your left palm for three seconds. Then press the thumb of your left hand into the center of your right palm for three seconds.

You are now ready to channel and direct divine energy onto the person you are praying with for healing.

The Healing Prayer of Moses

W E learn in Numbers 12 that Miriam, Moses's sister, was speaking ill of her brother. She went to her other brother, Aaron, to enlist his aid in her critique of Moses. Miriam committed the sin of *lashon hara* — "evil tongue," or slanderous speech — and was punished with the disease of *tzora'at,* leprosy, the classic punishment for *lashon hara.* Here we see the holistic nature of Judaism. The diseased soul of Miriam, which incited her to slanderous gossip, was manifested in her physical disease.

When Moses saw his sister's diseased body, he didn't rejoice in her suffering. Rather, he stretched out his arms and hands to receive God's healing light for her. He was an empty vessel to be filled with God's Holy Spirit. He was all forgiveness and love. This greatest of all people could see himself only as an empty vessel for what God decided to put into him. His humility and ability to forgive establish him as the greatest of all Jewish prophets.

We need to see ourselves as Moses saw himself, as an empty vessel, receiving only what God decides to give us. The great Kabbalistic secret here is that we do not do the healing, it is God who heals through us. You may memorize and internalize and practice the healing prayer of Moses, or any other healing prayer. It won't work unless you are extremely kind to people and greatly generous to others with time and money.

If you step on someone in the slightest way on your climb to the highest levels of spirituality, you are interfering in another person's purpose on this planet. This is what Miriam tried to do to Moses. She could not understand why God did not recognize her prophetic skills as much as He embraced the prophetic nature of Moses. So she tried to damage Moses with gossip, but it backfired.

I know I repeat myself, but to do these healing prayers effectively, it is crucially important that you spend alone time with God every day — and I don't mean five or ten minutes. You need to develop an ongoing prayerful relationship with God.

In *This Is for Everyone,* I shared Moses's healing prayer, *El Na Rifa Na La.* Subsequently, I learned from Rabbi Yaakov how to increase its voltage. The prayer as outlined in my first book can deliver wonderful results, and now I also want to share what Rabbi Yaakov taught me about it.

First let's review the original healing prayer of Moses as Rabbi Dan Dresher taught it to me. Then I will offer some of Rabbi Yaakov's alternative prayers that bring in the *Sefirot* and breathing techniques to increase its voltage. His methodologies are different than that of the original healing prayer, but are clearly based on a thorough knowledge of how it appears in Numbers 12.

When Rabbi Dan Dresher first introduced me to this prayer in Numbers 12, he described how Moses's faith and love for Miriam and God brought healing to his sister. Then he turned to the book of Exodus, where Moses spreads forth his hands in prayer (Exodus 9:33). That's when he taught me (as described in Chapter 10) to stretch forth my arms to the heavens when I pray for healing, with my palms facing upwards, and imagine two columns of bright light coming down from the heavens into my hands. As you may recall, he said to concentrate with *kavvanah* on the two columns of light, feeling the warmth of the light on the palms and fingers of my hands. As I visualize the two columns of light, I should know that I am making contact with the Divine Presence, and concentrate on bringing blessings down from above. (*Note:* Before you lift up your hands to God and receive the two columns of light, it is helpful to do one of the candle meditations in which you fill yourself up with God's light.)

Rabbi Dan taught me how to pour this healing light on the person I'm praying for. If the individual has an injured leg, for example, I should pour God's light on his leg, filling it with light, knowing that I am a vehicle of God's power and imaging my parishioner's leg well and healed. If I am praying with someone with cancerous lesions on his liver, I would pour light on his liver, filling his liver with light, while knowing that I am a channel for God's power, visualizing the light melting away the lesions.

Then I would say five times, *El Na Rifa Na La,* the same prayer that Moses prayed for his sister Miriam.

He taught Peggy and me that when we do the prayer, we should think as the Baal Shem Tov taught: We should pray as if God has already answered our prayer. We should pray in the Greater Mind. We are to visualize the person we are praying for as completely healed. We are to offer thanks to God for the person's healing even before he or she visits a doctor or gets an X-ray, because we know with faith and with the Greater Mind that healing has already happened. We knew all this when we were doing the prayer with two columns of light.

Rabbi Yaakov Dresher later taught me to include another column in this visualization. He said that there should be a middle column coming down from the heavens onto *Keter* on my head. This middle column of light constantly replenishes the light that I pour onto the individual for healing.

This chapter offers several "how to" healing prayers. Some appear difficult, and they are. But if you practice and do them regularly for several weeks, you can become very good at this process, and the healing results can be very great. You don't need to be a rabbi, a minister, or a priest to do these healing meditations wonderfully well. You need to love God, trust God, and practice. And then practice more. And then practice more. Practice, practice, practice, and you can be a wonderful instrument of God's healing.

HOW TO: Original Healing Prayer of Moses with Modifications

1. Recollect your morning prayers. Remember how you and God were brought together this morning. Recollect the candle meditation or any other meditation you did this morning, uniting you with God. The person for whom you are praying begins the healing session by sitting next to you.

2. Begin to say repeatedly with your eyes closed and with mounting energy this meditative prayer derived from Psalms 27:1 and 30:2.
     The Lord is my strength
     The Lord is my life
     The Lord is my light
     The Lord is my healing.

3. As you repeatedly say this out loud, you will begin to feel a mounting energy. The room will feel full of God's healing energy. When it does, stand and stretch out your arms at about eye level, with your palms turned up and your fingers pointing away from you. Try to feel two columns of light coming down from the heavens, one into each of your hands. Concentrate and visualize the light. Also visualize a third beam of light coming down from the heavens onto the *Sefira* of *Keter* on the crown of your head. This light will replenish the light which you will deliver with both hands to the person being healed. Know that this light constantly delivers God's healing light through your hands onto and into the person.

   Remember that prayer is an art, and that this visualization takes practice. With practice and experience and time, you will feel heat in your hands and on the crown of your head. When you see the light and feel the heat on your palms, turn your palms to face the person that needs healing. Pour this light on the person's entire body. Then pour the light on the specific part or parts of that person's body that need healing, heart or lungs or leg, or whatever it may be.

4. Concentrate on your love for God, God's love for you, and the love you have for the person you are praying for. You cannot hold resentment for that person. Nor can he or she hold resentment for you.

5. Continue to feel the light in your hands shining on and into the other person and say Moses's healing prayer in Hebrew five times. The Hebrew letters and words have mystical powers.

אל נא רפא נא לה

El Na Rifa Na La   El Na Rifa Na La   El Na Rifa Na La
El Na Rifa Na La   El Na Rifa Na La

O God, heal (person's name) now.

6. As you continue to pour God's light on and into the person, say personal prayers from your heart that you feel connect you to God. As you pray, concentrate on how much you are connected to God and how much you are connected to the person you are praying for.

7. See the person completely healed, doing some activity that he or she can only do when well. Know that the person is healed and say, "Oh give thanks to the Lord for He is Good, for His healing continues every day." And say with perfect faith, as you know the healing has taken place, "Thank you God for having healed (person's name)."

Say this healing prayer with faith and belief that it is working right now, as you say these words. Belief is of utmost importance. Without belief, without faith, without a heightened consciousness, prayer has little chance of working.

―――――――

As mentioned earlier, it was after Melinda Stengel and I finished *This Is for Everyone* that I began to work and study with Rabbi Yaakov Dresher. He taught me several alternate forms of this prayer. Through the years, I have seen that while some people respond very well to the original prayer of Moses above, others respond better to one or more of its alternate forms.

I remember asking Rabbi Yaakov why this is so. He said, "The same reason why some people respond to one medical treatment over another." He explained that the original Healing Prayer of Moses, though excellent, sometimes needs to be modified and sometimes even its modality needs to be changed, because every individual is unique and responds differently to prayer. Every person's soul is at a different level. He also explained clearly that the person who receives the prayer has to be a willing and embracing vessel. If a person strongly rejects the idea of God, healing and regular prayer, or strongly refuses to live the good life by regularly giving *tzedakah* and sharing with others — all this can greatly impede healing.

Rabbi Yaakov then asked if I knew where the idea of holding one's hands up in prayer originated. I recalled that we find Moses lifting up his hands in prayer to abate the plague of hail. Moses says in Exodus 9:29, "As soon as I am gone out of the city, I will spread forth my hands unto the Lord," and in verse 33, he does just that.

Also, when the ancient Israelites fought with the Amalekites in the desert, our text says, "And it came to pass when Moses held up his hand, Israel prevailed. But when he put down his hand, Amalek would prevail. When Moses's hands became heavy . . . Aaron and Hur lifted up his hands — one on one side, and the other on the other side. And Moses's hands were filled with faith until sunset" (Exodus 17:11–12). Rashi comments on this text that "filled with faith" means Moses continued to pray and had faith in God as his hands were held up high.

Rabbi Yaakov then gave me a Kabbalistic interpretation to this verse found in the *Zohar*: "When a man raises his hands in prayer, he directs his fingers toward the heavens."

I asked, "Hand or hands?"

The rabbi said, "Let's read on."

And sure enough, we say that the *Zohar* teaches that it means "hands." And furthermore, Rabbi Yaakov explained, when he raises his hands, his ten fingers are meant to signify the unification of the ten *Sefirot*.

Rabbi Yaakov then took from his bookshelf the *Tikkunei Ha-Zohar* and read, "Happy is the man who knows how to raise his will to the realms above, for his mouth utters names and his fingers write mysteries." It was then that he taught me that the intention behind raising the hands and fingers in prayer this way is to unify the ten *Sefirot*. We went over again the *Mishna* that has us identify the five masculine *Sefirot* as on the right hand and the five feminine *Sefirot* as on the left hand. When we lift up our hands at chest level, he explained — focusing on the ten *Sefirot*, five opposite five — we activate God's divine energy. And this energy can be used in Moses's healing prayer.

Rabbi Hezekiah's Healing Prayer

Rabbi Yaakov then showed me an amazing passage, a teaching from the great Rabbi Hezekiah on the *Zohar*. Rabbi Hezekiah says: "If one lifts and spreads his hands in prayer, the hands receive blessings from above, and the ten Powers or *Sefirot* concealed in the ten fingers will receive the blessings of above from God and deliver them to the person that is being blessed." It is important that when someone lifts up his hands to the heavens to activate the *Sefirotic* energies in the ten fingers, he must do so with *kavvanah* or with the intention of activating the ten *Sefirot* in his ten fingers. *This internal dynamic is a key secret of Kabbalistic healing.* When a person spreads out his hands and lifts them up in prayer, he unites the ten *Sefirot* and unites the name of God; the full name of God is a composite of all the *Sefirot* from *Keter* to *Malchut*, so that God's Holy Name is blessed from all sides. This unifying of the ten *Sefirot* in prayer adds tremendous metaphysical power to the prayer.

Rabbi Yaakov then introduced me to a mystical commentary on the Torah in which Rabbi Bachya ben Asher interprets Exodus 17:11, the verse that describes when, during their exodus in the desert from Egypt, the ancient Israelites were attacked by the Amalekites. "And it came to pass, when Moses held up his hand, that Israel prevailed. And when he let down his hand, Amalek prevailed."

Rabbi Bachya teaches that when Moses raised his hands toward the heavens, he concentrated on his ten fingers, which were pointed "at the heights of the heavens." In raising his hands, Moses did something very similar to what the ancient Jewish priests did when they raised their hands to bless people. When they concentrated on the number ten, they would focus on the ten *Sefirot*, the ten Divine powers within the soul of God. When the priest stretched forth his arms, with the fingers and thumb of each hand identifying with the appropriate *Sefirot*, his palms were facing upward so that the blessing of energy would flow into each finger separately.

Rabbi Yaakov then taught me a more powerful Mosaic healing prayer, focusing on the ten *Sefirot* of God's soul, which of course manifests in our own soul.

HOW TO: An Alternate Healing Prayer of Moses with the *Sefirot*

1. Sit in a comfortable chair in a comfortable place, with your back upright. If possible, loosen your pants or unbuckle your belt. The person you are praying for should be seated comfortably next to you.

2. Recollect the prayers and/or meditations you did at home this morning that united you with God.

3. Begin to say repeatedly with eyes closed and with mounting energy this meditative prayer derived from Psalms 27:1 and 30:2:

   The Lord is my strength
   The Lord is my life
   The Lord is my light
   The Lord is my healing.

4. Put your hands in front of you fifteen inches apart and identify the five masculine *Sefirot* with the five fingers of the right hand and the five feminine *Sefirot* with the five fingers of the left hand. As you imagine the *Sefirot* corresponding to the five fingers of each hand, you are polarizing these *Sefirot* and creating strong spiritual tension. This tension is the divine energy within you.

5. Now stand and stretch forward your arms, turning your palms at eye level to face the heavens. Try to feel two columns of gold/white light coming down from the heavens, one column of light going into the palm of each hand. Also, feel a third column of gold/white light coming from heaven into *Keter* at the crown of your head; this will replenish the light you pour on the person you are praying for.

6. Feel the light spread into each finger and be conscious that on your right hand, the thumb is filled with *Keter* light, the index finger is filled with *Chochma* light, the middle finger is filled with *Chesed* light, the ring finger is filled with *Tiferet* light, and the little finger is filled with *Netzach* light. On the left hand, the thumb is filled with *Bina* light, the index finger is filled with *Gevurah* light, the middle finger is filled with *Hod* light, the ring finger is filled with *Yesod* light, and the little finger is filled with *Malchut* light. Look at the illustration below.

   With your hands facing upward, feel God's light not only in your palms, but also in each finger, and silently identify the *Sefirot* on each hand. Feel the light and the heat, and remember that you are channeling God's Light — for just as God is made up of the *Sefirot*, so are you.

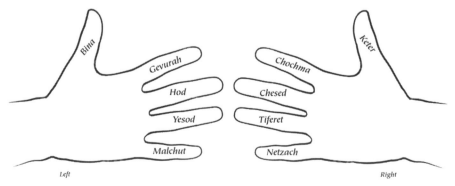

7. When you see God's Light with your mind's eye and feel the heat, turn your palms to face the person that needs healing. Pour the light on the person's entire body. Then, pour this light on any part of his or her body that needs healing — perhaps it's the heart or lungs or liver. As you do this, also see ten threads of gold/white light — five issuing from the fingers of the right hand and five issuing from the fingers of the left. As you pour this light, remember that you are bringing God's healing light to this person who needs healing.

8. Mentally identify the ten *Sefirot* on your ten fingers. Pour the two columns of light / ten threads of light from your palms onto and into the individual and the specific organ that needs healing. By doing this, you are identifying with God and also identifying the person who is being healed with God. You both are becoming one with God as the healing is taking place.

9. Concentrate on your love for God, God's love for you, and the love you have for the person you are praying for. You are all one with God.

10. Say *El Na Rifa Na La* five times in Hebrew and then in English, *O God, heal _____ now.* Say this healing prayer with faith and belief that it is working now.

11. As you continue to pour light on the person, say personal prayers in your own words and feel the love you have for this person.

12. See the person you are praying for completely healed, doing some activity that he/she can only do when well. Know that the person is healed, and say, *Thank you God* (or *Hashem*) *for having healed _____.* Or you might want to say, *Hodu l'Adonai kee tov kee l'Olam chasdo,* or in English, *Give thanks to the Lord for He is good, for His healing continues every day.*

Helpful hints to make this prayer even more powerful

When you receive divine energy, God's *Ru'ach*, into the palms and fingers of each hand — five masculine energies and five feminine energies, plus energy in each palm — your tongue becomes the place where the spiritual tension mentioned earlier builds up. By tongue here, we mean speech. Your speech, that is, your healing prayer, your words, will be able to activate powerfully these ten energies of God.

To do this, you will want to visualize God's energy flowing in you as ten threads of light while you verbally articulate (with your *tongue*, of course) a prayer like *El Na Rifa Na La*. Doing this activates God's *Ru'ach* so it becomes *Ru'ach HaKodesh*, God's Holy *Ru'ach*. Proper speech activates the power of the healing energies.

With this added element of technique, when you lift your arms up toward the heavens, you not only concentrate on the number ten, you also say to yourself (or whisper quietly) the Hebrew names of the different *Sefirot*. When you pour God's energy onto the person or the affected organ, you focus on each individual *Sefira*'s energy in your hands and say each name silently or in a whisper. Understand that your ten fingers represent the ten *Sefirot* — indeed they *are* the ten *Sefirot*. This increases the spiritual force. The raised hands, the focus on each *Sefira*, the silent naming of each one, pouring these ten lights simultaneously on the person's affected organ or body, speaking an appropriate prayer from your heart and soul — all these together increase the power of the prayer exponentially.

Remember, these ten spiritual powers receive God's blessing from above and bless the person who is making the healing prayer. In other words, the *Sefirotic* energies from above are what activate their *Sefirotic* counterpart energies in the person who is doing the healing prayer.

Another powerful meditation based on the prayer of Moses is to lift *Adonai* out of Her exile and bring Her together with Her male consort, as discussed in the Preface of this book, and demonstrated in Chapter 7.

HOW TO: An Alternate Healing Prayer of Moses with *Sefirot* and Balancing Male and Female Divine Energies in Every Cell

In the beginning, this alternate prayer using both *Sefirotic* fingers and male/female divine energies is difficult; but if you practice it often, the difficulties will cease and slip away. It will come naturally. You can let your intuition guide you. Sometimes my intuition emphasizes uniting male and female divine energies, sometimes it emphasizes *Sefirotic* energies of the fingers only. Mostly, I do both male/female healing energies and *Sefirotic* finger energies, and the results are very positive. Work hard, pray a lot, and practice, and these meditations will bring phenomenal results.

1–4. In your *mi'at meekdash,* repeat steps 1–4 from the Alternate Healing Prayer of Moses with the *Sefirot* meditation above.

5. Stand and stretch forward your arms, turning your palms at eye level to face the heavens. Try to feel two columns of light coming down from the heavens into the palms of each hand. Feel a column of light coming from heaven into *Keter* at the crown of your head, replenishing the light which you are pouring on the person you are praying for. Visualize in each of the columns many sets of the holy letters *YHVH* יהוה in purple characters.

6. Feel the light spread from the palms into each finger and be conscious that on your right hand, the right thumb is filled with *Keter* light, the index finger is filled with *Chochma* light, the middle finger is filled with *Chesed* light, the ring finger is filled with *Tiferet* light, and the little finger is filled with *Netzach* light. On the left hand, the left thumb is filled with *Bina* light, the index finger is filled with *Gevurah* light, the middle finger is filled with *Hod* light, the ring finger is filled with *Yesod* light, and the little finger is filled with *Malchut* light (see page 158).

   With your hands facing upward, feel God's light not only in your palms, but in each finger and silently identify the *Sefirot* on each hand. Feel the light and feel the heat, and remember that you are channeling God's Light, for just as God is made up of the *Sefirot,* so are you.

7. When you see God's Light with your mind's eye and feel the heat, turn your hands to face the person who needs healing. Visualize every cell in that person's body filled with the feminine divine energies of the *Shechina* or *Alef Daled Nun Yod* אדני in green characters. When every cell has only female divine energies, this leads to imbalance. For health to arise, every cell also needs male divine energies, *YHVH* יהוה which we visualize in purple characters, so that each cell of each organ has divine male and divine female energies in balance: יאהדונהי. To bring about this balance, you need to direct *YHVH* יהוה male energies into each organ that needs healing and into every cell of the person's body. So you direct *YHVH* יהוה male energies into the affected organ or body part and into the whole body: Pour the light that is filled with purple sets of *YHVH* יהוה on

that person's heart or lungs or liver — on any part of the body that needs healing. As you pour this light, know that you are a channel for God's healing light to this person who needs healing.

8. When you have visualized and activated one cell in alternating purple and green characters יאהדונהי *Yod Alef Hey Daled Vav Nun Hey Yod*, know intuitively that all the cells have embraced this balance of alternating male/female divine energy.

9. By recognizing that your ten fingers represent the ten *Sefirot* and your raised hands identify with God, you are now able to bring balance to one cell and identify with the person who is being healed by God. God and the person being healed are all becoming one with God and healing is taking place.

10. Concentrate on your love for God, God's love for you, and the love you have for the person you are praying for. For you are both one with God.

11. Say *El Na Rifa Na La* five times in Hebrew and then say one time in English, *O God, heal (person's name) now*. Know that it is working *now*.

12. As you continue to pour light on the person, say personal prayers in your own words and feel the love you have for this person.

13. See the person you are praying for completely healed, doing some activity that he/she can only do when well. Know that the person is healed, and say, *Thank you God* (or *Hashem*) *for having healed (person's name)*. Or, you might want to say, *Hodu l'Adonai kee tov kee l'Olam chasdo*, which means: *Give thanks to the Lord for He is good, for His healing continues every day.*

Left Hand/Right Hand Modality

Rabbi Yaakov also taught me how to use the *Sefirotic* columns in a different way for healing prayer. In this modality, your left hand receives divine energy, which is transformed within you, while your right hand delivers this transformed healing energy into the person being healed. Even if you are left-handed, you still need to adhere to the Kabbalistic principle that the left hand receives and the right hand delivers.

I use this left hand/right hand approach to healing about as often as the two-hands-giving-while-receiving-from-*Keter* modality. Both approaches are equally good. When I practice distance healing, I almost always use the two-handed approach.

HOW TO: Kabbalistic Left Hand/Right Hand Healing Prayer

As you remember from our study of the Kabbalistic tree, the left column is feminine, the left arm and left hand are feminine, which receives, always receives. The right column of the tree, the right arm and right hand, are masculine, which always delivers. Kabbalists developed the left hand/right hand delivery system into a true healing modality. Here you see the Kabbalistic idea of the left part of the tree and the right part of the tree working together.

1. Sit in a comfortable chair in a comfortable place, with your back upright. If possible, loosen your clothing. The person you are praying for should be seated comfortably next to you.

2. Recollect the prayers and/or meditations you did this morning uniting you with God.

3. Say repeatedly with eyes closed and with mounting energy the following meditative prayer derived from Psalms 27:1 and 30:2:

   The Lord is my strength
   The Lord is my life
   The Lord is my light
   The Lord is my healing.

4. Say Rabbi Nachman's blessing: "Our God and God of our fathers, bless me and bless my hands, that I might become a pure instrument of Your healing light, so that Your healing/light energy flows through me, and through my hands, bringing complete healing to the person I am praying for." Focus on being an instrument of God, receiving and delivering God's light/energy.

5. Stretch out both your arms with palms and fingers facing upward. Imagine God's light entering both hands. Focus on the number ten, remembering that your ten fingers are receiving the divine energy of the *Sefirot*. This is the Kabbalistic secret of the ten fingers. Feel the energy and be able to recognize the *Sefirot* on your right and left fingers as indicated on page 158.

6. Keep your left hand with left palm and fingers facing upward. Imagine God's light/energy entering into your left hand, fingers and palms, with the palm of your right hand facing the affected area of the individual that needs to be healed. Visualize *Sefirotic* light/energy leaving the right hand — both the right palm and the right fingers.

7. Your focus now should be on the energies of your left and right hands, the palms and fingers. Focus on the *Sefirotic* energies of your left hand. Stare at the left hand with its five fingers, feeling the *Sefirotic* energies in the palm and fingers. Do this for about one minute. Then stare at the right hand and its *Sefirotic* energies, while facing the individual you are praying for. Your focus should be on God's Light/Energy entering your left hand and leaving the right hand.

8. Before you place your right hand over the affected organ of the person you are praying for, gently rotate the wrist of your right hand in counterclockwise motion over the person's body; as you do this visualize God's light entering your left hand, leaving your right hand, and filling his/her body organs. Then do a general prayer that this person's respiratory system and circulatory system and skeletal system and digestive system are all in harmony with each other, that everything is in balance.

9. After perhaps one or two minutes, focus the energies of your right hand over the affected organ. Concentrate on divine light entering your left hand, being transformed by the *Sefirot* of the left hand, being passed as so transformed over to the right hand, being further transformed by the *Sefirot* of the right hand, and then leaving the right hand. As mentioned earlier, when God's *Ru'ach* or light/energy has been transformed by your ten *Sefirot* in this way, it becomes *Ru'ach HaKodesh,* sacred energy or holy spirit.

10. Visualize the affected organ or limb filled with this holy light. Healing is taking place. As you continue to visualize healing take place, recite *El Na Rifa Na La* five times.

11. Now recite a personal prayer from your own soul or heart. Be passionate. Pray for your friend.

12. See your friend completely healed, doing some activity he/she could not do while ill. Thank God for healing him or her.

A few years ago, our friends Scott and Ivy Kroman went with us for an extended weekend trip to New York City. Just a day after we arrived, Scott experienced great pain and swelling in his knee when we were out. I chose to do the left hand/right hand Kabbalistic healing prayer to remove his pain and swelling, because I thought that lifting both arms with palms upward to the heavens where we were might have landed me in Bellevue Hospital's psychiatric ward. When I shared this concern with my wife, she said, "Douglas, where's your faith? This is the city where the Naked Cowboy walks around. Do you really think anyone would look at you twice?"

I heard her, but I still opted for left hand/right hand modality prayer. And here is the story in Scott Kroman's words:

> We arrived in New York City, ready to have many great meals and see some wonderful Broadway shows. The next morning we awoke, and my knee was swollen three times the normal size. I could hardly move. The pain was excruciating. I had a hard time getting my pants on over my knee. We met for breakfast at a beautiful café and were seated by the window, facing the street. I spoke of my problem — how am I going to do New York?
>
> Rabbi Doug said calmly, "Don't worry. Prayer has worked before. It will work again." Rabbi Doug got down on one knee, as though he was proposing to me. The front of his body faced towards me, his back was towards the street.
>
> I sat back, relaxed as Rabbi placed his hand in front of my knee. Rabbi said, "Dear God, we came on this journey together. We can't leave Scott behind in pain." Silently he prayed, and I felt the sensation of heat flowing through my knee . . . I felt the pain go away. Thank you God once again. The swelling went away, the knee became painless. We left the restaurant to adventure in the streets of New York City.

Both Rabbi Dan and Rabbi Yaakov Dresher always emphasized how important it is for me and for the person with me to understand that we are created in the image of God. Not only that, but if I want the prayer to succeed, I must realize that we are filled with the Presence of God. The vision that I have of the Presence of God should be a vision of light, filling me from head to toe, filling my chest cavity, my arms, my fingers, my legs, my toes. This vision, in part, comes from my many prayers and meditations done at home that morning.

Years ago, a mechanic who was taking a class with me encouraged me to think of the human body as an energy system such as a battery. He asked me to imagine placing a wrench across the poles of an automobile battery — an experiment he often did with high school senior classes that he taught. When you do that, the wrench melts. Then in the class he would attach the wires of an FM radio to the poles. He asked if I knew what would happen. I answered, "No idea."

He said that he received symphonic music. He said the class picked up waves coming from a great distance, and explained that the difference between the wrench and the radio is not the *energy* but the *circuitry* through which the energy flows.

When we do healing work, we are like the battery. From the Kabbalistic perspective, God's energy, which is everywhere, is transformed by the different *Sefirot* of which we are made. We are like the battery with different built in transformers, *Sefirot,* that draw in and hold and release that energy. When we meditate, we are connecting our trillions and trillions of cells in our body to the Great Mechanic — God. When we do this, our *Sefirot* become activated, which allows for the divine flow in every cell. And the divine experience that we have is the circuitry through which this energy flows, when raised to divine energy.

I would like to close this chapter with a wonderful insight into the prayer we have been discussing that one of Rabbi Yaakov's students recently shared with me. He first showed me that the Prayer of Moses, *El Na Rifa Na La,* has eleven Hebrew letters. He then pointed out that when Moses asked God for His Name at the Burning Bush, God replied, אהיה אשר אהיה *Ehyeh asher Ehyeh* (also eleven letters): "I am Who I am." Or, "I am."

Since seeing this, when I pray for someone's injured limb or organ and say out loud, *El Na Rifa Na La,* I also visualize the eleven-letter prayer *Ehyeh asher Ehyeh* on the injured person's organ. It is not a coincidence that the name of God and Moses's prayer both have eleven letters. In my opinion, it shows that these mystical phrases are strongly related. I find combining them in this way to be very inspiring and efficacious.

Rabbi Nachman and Breath

KABBALISTIC breathing corresponds to the continuous vibrations of everything in the universe. Everything is in constant vibration because everything is made up of the *Sefirot,* and the energies of the *Sefirot* are in constant vibration. There is no rest in the universe. From the smallest atom to the largest planet, there is movement and vibration. If a tiny atom would cease to vibrate, the equilibrium and universal balance would be thrown off.

When we study and practice Kabbalistic healing, we immediately recognize that the atoms of the human body continuously vibrate and its cells are constantly created, destroyed, replaced, and changed. When we base Kabbalistic healing on breathing techniques, we also recognize the crucial importance of a free-flowing rhythm. The rhythmic breathing that we practice in healing corresponds to the rhythmic breathing of the universe.

Everything in the universe functions rhythmically, and this is what keeps it alive. We see this with our rhythmic heartbeat and, of course, we see this with breathing. Rhythmic breathing is the very foundation of Kabbalistic healing. Illness occurs when we have a collapse of this rhythmic behavior of the body or cells. Healing occurs when a cell returns to its functional purpose, to participate in rhythmic pulsation. Kabbalah teaches us that whether we get sick on a physical, mental, or spiritual level, sickness begins at the cellular level. For health to occur, the cell must return to its original state of rhythmic pulsation.

For a sick cell to be healthy, it must return to the state it was in before illness caused a corruption in its spiritual DNA. The DNA-like forces are the physical form and sound vibrations of the Hebrew letters. These twenty-two letters have creative power. These twenty-two energy forces became the DNA life-forces behind the entire cosmos.

We need to see the Hebrew letters encoded in a prayer as spiritual software. This is crucial if healing prayer is to have not only meaning but also efficacy. When *YHVH* appears in a prayer, we need to recognize that — as is the case with the *Sh'ma* — we cannot think of that prayer in a conventional way. We must recognize that these Hebrew DNA forces are codes that allow us to connect the divine principle within us to the divine principle outside of us.

If we are unwell, we need to recognize that *YHVH* is not a symbol *representing* God, but a code that allows us to *connect* the divine within to the divine without and thereby effect healing. This is a great Kabbalistic secret of healing: Prayer, and specifically healing prayer, is not a mumbo jumbo of words making supplication before a deity. It is our effort to identify the inner God, within us, with the outer God outside of us — or the small "I" with the greater "I," *YHVH*. And we do this by practicing prayer and meditation rhythmically.

When I begin healing prayer with an individual, I usually spend six months to a year praying with her once a week. I also teach her family members or close friends to do this prayer with her, so that she can have a prayer partner. This *chevruta* style of praying allows the person who is ill to know she is not alone. It also reinforces the methodology so she won't keep worrying if she got it "right" from me. But most importantly, one who is ill and in pain needs someone full of faith who sees the world optimistically and sees her completely healed.

A healing meditation that I find very effective is a breathing meditation that uses the DNA forces of *YHVH*. As mentioned earlier, this sequence of energy forces is so strong that Kabbalists call it the *Tetragrammaton* or Face of God.

HOW TO: Breathing Meditation with *YHVH* Forces

    1. I ask the person I'm praying with to start by visualizing the Hebrew letters *YHVH* יהוה in their mind's eye. Visualize each letter very large. See each letter as a black character, as it appears in the prayer book. See each letter very large, so large that it engulfs you. First

visualize the *Yod* י, then the *Hey* ה, then the *Vav* ו, then the *Hey* ה until the complete *Tetragrammaton* of *YHVH* is before you.

2. As you focus on God's face in this way, breathe in gently and deeply through your nostrils and then exhale. Do this rhythmic breathing six times while visualizing the *Tetragrammaton* יהוה.

3. Now it's time to become one with *YHVH* יהוה, to identify the Face of God within you with the Face of God outside of you. Visualize the *Yod* this time filled with white light. As you breathe in deeply through your nostrils, visualize the *Yod* entering the *Chochma* and *Bina* parts of your forehead, or the Third Eye. Feel the healing warmth of the *Yod* within your head.

4. Now exhale through your nostrils. As you do this, feel the *Hey* shining with white light throughout your being. Know that as you exhale, you are releasing all impurities and illness from your spiritual system.

5. Now visualize the *Vav* filled with white warm light and inhale through your nostrils. As you inhale, feel the *Vav* entering your whole body, energizing you and healing you. Continue to feel the *Vav* radiating throughout you.

6. As you exhale, feel that your body is being healed by the final *Hey* in white light, filling every cell in your body. Notice the rhythmic breathing of inhaling and exhaling, inhaling and exhaling.

7. Repeat this process twenty-five times, for a total of twenty-six times all together. Remember, inhale on *Yod*, exhale on *Hey*, inhale on *Vav*, exhale on *Hey*. Do it all rhythmically. As you inhale and exhale these energy forces, try to silently hear the sound of them. This is important. As you breathe in the different letters, hear in your mind the sound of each one. We want to correlate the sound of the letter with its visual image.

The *gematria* of the *Tetragrammaton* is 26:
Yod = 10   *Hey* = 5   *Vav* = 6   *Hey* = 5, for a total of 26.
Thus, our mystics encourage us to do this spiritual prayer of inhaling and exhaling the letters twenty-six times.

What we are doing in this process is identifying with the Supreme Origin of all creation. The *Tetragrammaton*, the blueprint of all existence, is an amazing energy force, since its four Hebrew letters are associated with all the supernal worlds and with the Tree of Life. The Tree of Life contains within it the perfection and healing before we devolved into the domain of the Tree of Knowledge, with its duality of health and illness, living and dying.

As we learned from the Law of Correspondence, whatever is true on one level of reality has a corresponding truth on every other level. The relationships between the macrocosm and the microcosm, the sun, the planets, and the atoms all follow rhythmic laws. The celestial bodies and the bodies of Adam and Eve's descendants are subject to this law. So is the transformation of *Ru'ach* into *Ru'ach HaKodesh*.

When we understand and practice rhythmic breathing, we become a pure channel for transforming *Ru'ach* into *Ru'ach HaKodesh*. The transformation happens through recognizing and practicing *kavvanah* with rhythmic breathing. The Kabbalist can increase the flow of circulation and can maintain control of the autonomic nervous system by using *kavvanah* with rhythmic breathing. The Kabbalist is able to serve the purpose of healing by bringing into his or her body a great amount of *Ru'ach* and transforming it into *Ru'ach HaKodesh*.

My studies with Rabbi Yaakov also brought me to recognize the holiness and power of another Hebrew name for God, *Yah*. *Yah* has the numerical value of 15, which suggests a meaning we can translate into a Kabbalistic rule for breathing. This rule for rhythmic breathing, based on the holy name of *Yah*, is that the units of inhalation and exhalation should be the same. That is, six inhalations and six exhalations, while the units for retention between breaths should be half that number.

Moses ben Jacob Cordovero (1522–1570), one of the greatest Kabbalists ever to teach and preach in the Holy Land, used many breathing techniques in his holy meditations. Another great Kabbalist, Abraham ben Samuel Abulafia (1240–1291 *ca.*), also stressed the importance of breathing when one wants to identify with the Spirit of God. His meditative breathing techniques fill many volumes of his ancient classic works.

The Hebrew letters we use in prayers are not only sacred, they are mystical. Each has a soul and is an instrument of a different kind of energy that God uses to create. Recall how the *Sefer Yetzirah* says God creates the universe. "There are twenty-two foundation letters. He (God) engraved them. He carved them. He weighed them. He combined them.

He permuted them. And He formed with them the soul of all that was created and the soul of all that will be created."[1] When we study this text and its commentaries mystically, we recognize that we humans need not use the Hebrew language for communication only; we also can use it for creative purposes such as healing.

Rabbi Yaakov repeated many times enthusiastically what Rabbi Dan Dresher had taught me years before: that since the world is created again and again every day by the Hebrew letters, and since it continues to be sustained by this divine language, *then the laws of language are identical to the laws of the universe.* This is a deep Kabbalistic secret that we use in healing. And when we investigate and study the nature and energies of each of the Hebrew letters, we can better understand human nature.

So, we learn that the Hebrew letters are alive, and that they are related to the organs and vessels of the human body. When we understand these relationships between them and the body's organs and limbs, we can see why we use them in healing prayer.

Rabbi Yaakov and I also discussed the following text from *Sefer Yetzirah*:

> Twenty-two foundation letters:
>
> He engraved them with voice,
>
> He carved them with breath (*Ru'ach*),
>
> He set them in the mouth (*Peh/Dibbur*).[2]

He was teaching me a healing technique which derives from this *Mishna*, that we engrave with voice, then carve with breath as we meditate on the Hebrew letters. We concentrate on the breath that is exhaled while we pronounce the letters. In the end, we speak the letter. So the three stages through which an utterance is manifest are: *Kol, Ru'ach, Dibbur* — sound, breath, and speech.

In Kabbalistic language, the rate of vibration of the letter that happens when it is spoken with proper breathing techniques is called *Kol*.

Breathing Meditations

The meditative healing exercise based on the left and right hand columns of the Tree of Life that we learned earlier (pages 162-164) is quite powerful in itself. It is even more powerful when combined with rhythmic breathing. In the healing meditations below, breath is a key theme. *Nishimah*, the Hebrew word for breath, is spelled with the same letters as *Neshamah*, the Hebrew word for soul. In doing these meditations, we literally re-enact the verse from Genesis 2:7 which teaches, "Then the Lord formed man of the dust of the ground, breathing into his nostrils the breath of life; and man became a living soul." The text shows the relationship between the breath and soul, both words being identical.

When we do these exercises, we follow the Kabbalistic rule for rhythmic breathing based on the Holy name of *Yah* (*Yod-Hey*): that the unity of inhalation and exhalation should be the same — that is, six inhalations and six exhalations — while the units for retention between breaths should be half that number.

HOW TO: Healing Meditation Based on the Kabbalistic Tree of Life Using Rhythmic Breathing

1. Go to your *mi'at meekdash*. Sit comfortably, in a comfortable chair, with your back upright. If possible, unbuckle your belt or loosen your pants. The person you are praying for is seated comfortably next to you.

2. Recollect your morning prayers and meditations that brought you closer to God.

3. Extend your left arm at eye level with the left palm turned upward toward the heavens while your right palm or "projecting" hand faces the part or organ of your friend's body that needs healing, at a distance of about six inches or nearer.

4. With your left arm still extended and your palm facing upward, inhale gently and deeply through your nostrils, counting 1, 2, 3, 4, 5, 6. As you inhale, visualize God's *Ru'ach* healing/light/energy coming down through the heavens as a gold/white light into your palm.

5. Retain God's *Ru'ach* in the palm of your left hand, while holding your breath and counting 1, 2, 3. *Ru'ach* is being transformed in your palm to *Ru'ach HaKodesh* because of your intentionality.

6. As your right hand faces the diseased organ or limb, exhale through your nostrils while counting 1, 2, 3, 4, 5, 6 and visualizing God's gold/white *Ru'ach HaKodesh* light entering and transforming

the diseased organ and healing the diseased conditions.

7. Offer a prayer from your own heart and/or visualize *YHVH* יהוה on the diseased organ. I often visualize the *YHVH* in the ten colors of the *Sefirot* — translucent gold, white, green, baby blue, blood red, purple, dark pink, light pink, orange, and navy blue, one after another. This is based on Moses Cordovero's color system found in *Pardes Rimonim*.

8. Thank God for healing your friend, with the conviction that your friend has received God's healing. It is at this time that you visualize your friend well and healed. And again, you thank God with all your heart, soul and strength for this healing.

During the healing prayer, it is important to let God's *Ru'ach* pour into the person you are praying for, recognizing that you are merely the *Tzinor* or instrument, transforming God's *Ru'ach* to *Ru'ach HaKodesh*.

HOW TO: Alternate Version — Healing Meditation Based on the Kabbalistic Tree of Life Using Rhythmic Breathing

1–5. Repeat steps 1–5 above, with the change that the gold/white *Ru'ach* light is now filled with many sets of *YHVH* יהוה male transcendent divine energies in purple characters.

6. As your right hand faces the diseased organ or limb, exhale through your nostrils while counting 1, 2, 3, 4, 5, 6 and visualizing God's gold/white *Ru'ach HaKodesh* light, filled with purple sets of *YHVH* יהוה, entering and transforming the cells of the diseased organ. This light is entering every cell in the diseased organ so that the *Adonai* אדני female divine energies in green characters in each cell are lifted up from Her exile and joined to the male divine energies of *YHVH* יהוה.

7. Now visualize each cell with its divine female and male energies in balance, with יאהדונהי in alternating colors of purple and green. Male and female divine energies are in balance.

8. Offer a personal prayer asking God to continue to transform every cell in the diseased organ or limb to be healthy and strong, and to have male and female divine energies in balance. Please let God know how deeply you love the person you are praying for.

9. Visualize with full faith that the person you are praying for is

completely well . . . and remember always to be in the Greater Mind. Then, thank God for healing your friend. Know that you, your friend, and God are One — healthy, in balance, and free from disease.

I often use these two left hand/right hand Kabbalistic prayers with rhythmic breathing. Sometimes I use one, sometimes the other. You have to use your intuition to know which will be more effective with the particular person who needs God's healing. There are times when I combine parts of both prayers. For example, I might first visualize the *YHVH* in the ten colors of the *Sefirot*. Afterwards, I might see with my mind's eye ten sets of *YHVH*, all in purple characters, because purple represents healing. And then I would combine the male energies of the *YHVH* in purple characters with the female energies of *Adonai* in green characters to achieve balance of the male and female divine energies. This flexibility comes about through practice. The more you practice, the more you study, the more proficient you will become in this type of meditative blessing.

But again, no matter how proficient you are with technique, the blessings you want to deliver will not work if you don't live a life governed by spiritual law. You must constantly be aware that God is everywhere — not only in you or in the person you wish to bless. God is in the trees and plants and shrubs around you and in the walls of the room in which you do your meditative healing. You need to live each moment recognizing that God is One, which means we are all connected with the One God who sees and hears everything. You need to be the kindest, most generous, most loving person you can be to people and animals and to nature itself. This is enormously empowering.

When you are compassionate, generous, and loving to all beings, you activate the spiritual *tzinor* or pipeline that connects you to God. Then, only then, do your newly learned spiritual meditative techniques work. *Kindness is the key to healing. This is the single greatest secret to Kabbalistic healing.*

———

Last year I began praying with a middle-aged man who had cancerous lesions on his liver. He came to me because I have been his family's rabbi for almost ten years. Jeffrey was very skeptical, not only about healing prayer, but also about a God who is personally active in this world. He had difficulty accepting that the God of the universe is concerned about every person in this world. But since his medical prognosis was poor, and since he enjoyed my sermons, he decided to suspend his skepticism and go with the flow.

"Let's try this healing prayer and see what happens," he said to me one rainy morning.

"You know it is crucial that you have a prayer partner. I thought Amy was coming with you today."

"Well, I wanted to hear how this works before I commit myself to it."

I then proceeded to share with him the origin of the Mosaic healing prayer in Numbers 12 (See Chapter 11) and to explain the importance of having a prayer partner. Then I told Jeffrey this story from the Talmud *Berakhot* p. 5a.

Rabbi Chiya bar Abba was ill. Rabbi Yochanan went to visit him and asked him, "Are your sufferings dear to you?" Rabbi Chiya bar Abba answered him, "Neither they nor their reward." Rabbi Yochanan said, "Give me your hand." Rabbi Chiya bar Abba gave him his hand and Rabbi Yochanan revived him.

A similar incident took place when Rabbi Yochanan was ill. Rabbi Chanina went to visit him and asked, "Are these sufferings dear to you?" Rabbi Yochanan answered, "Neither they nor their reward." Rabbi Chanina said, "Give me your hand." Rabbi Yochanan gave him his hand and Rabbi Chanina revived him.

Then the Talmud asks, "Why did Rabbi Yochanan need Rabbi Chanina's help? Can't Rabbi Yochanan pray for himself?" The Talmud answers that "a captive cannot release himself from prison." This teaches that a person who is ill, suffering, and in pain, needs someone to pray for him or her. That person needs outside help.

This made sense to Jeffrey. At least enough sense that from the following week on, Jeffrey, his wife Amy, and I met regularly on Monday mornings to do healing prayer so that the cancerous lesions on his liver would diminish or even disappear.

The first week that Jeffrey brought Amy, I shared with them how to do the healing prayer of Moses. After two months, Jeffrey's MRI showed no decrease in the size of the lesions. His skepticism became stronger than his willingness to continue the prayer work. Even Amy, a woman of faith, grew sad at the prayer's apparent lack of efficacy.

I then decided to try an alternate version of the healing prayer of Moses, pointing my hands toward the heavens, uniting the *Sefirot* with my fingers and becoming a channel for God's healing energy. But, after a month of praying together this way each Monday, and Jeffrey praying at home with Amy every day, it appeared that his liver cancer was even more debilitating than it had been when he began seeing me. He was physically sick from radiation treatment, and he and Amy did not feel the Presence of God in their prayers at home. They said they felt God's Presence when they prayed together with me, but it was too difficult for them to feel it at home when they prayed together each day. They were finding it difficult to keep believing in God as Jeffrey's condition appeared to worsen.

I think they felt God's Presence with me because I always pray with my parishioners in front of the open Ark where we keep our Holy Scrolls, the Torah. It is breathtaking to see this and one can't help but be moved and inspired. Also, I have done healing prayers in front of the open Ark for more than thirty years. I believe the holiness and energy of the area is so strong that one can't help but feel the Divine Presence there. I have seen amazing things happen there. All the same Jeffrey was not getting better. So I flew to visit Rabbi Yaakov.

I joined Rabbi Yaakov for early morning *minyan* (prayer service), and afterwards we had some schnapps and herring before we drove to his home. We went into his study and, as soon as we sat down, I blurted out, "The healing prayer isn't working! I don't understand."

"Slow down Douglas. What do you mean, it's not working?"

I then explained that I had done the healing prayer in different ways yet my parishioner was getting worse, not better. "In addition to the healing prayer, does Jeffrey enjoy an inner spiritual life?" he said to me.

"Yes, he prays the *Amidah*[3] every day."

"What about his external life? Does he give to *tzedakah,* charity, for social justice? Does he act with kindness toward others? Does he feel worthy? Does he feel he deserves to be healed?"

"Yes to all those questions." I answered. Rabbi Yaakov then asked me to define the Hebrew term *Ru'ach*. I said, "It means wind, air, spirit, and breath. Sometimes God is called *Ru'ach HaKodesh,* the Holy Spirit or the Holy Breath."

"Good," he said, smiling. "And, what is breath?" he asked.

I answered that breath or *Ru'ach* includes the two opposite and alternate activities of inhaling and exhaling air . . . that it is through breathing that we become one with the world and God . . . that this is so because the air that fills every nook and cranny of the outside world enters our lungs and travels to every cell within our body . . . that it is through breathing that we enjoy life . . . more than that, breath is life, because breath is the bridge that connects us with the outside world. And I cited Genesis 2:7: "Then the Lord God formed man of the dust of the ground and *breathed* into his nostrils the *breath* of life; then man became a living soul."

Rabbi Yaakov then said, "If you sit and become aware of your breath, you will see that, really, you and the universe are one. When you are 'awake,' you will be 'aware' that the universe is breathing. Your lungs expand and contract, responding to the universe. Imagine the universe as a vast Being that is alive, and that you are a cell in this body. And you, the cell, are kept alive by the *Ru'ach* of the universe. In Ezekiel 36:26, we read, 'I will place a holy *Ru'ach* within you.' This *Ru'ach* is the Spirit of God that every living being inhales, this *Ru'ach* is our breath; and it is through breathing that we focus on the present and not the past or future. When we are in the NOW, we are alive, filled with the Breath of God. The past is gone, the future has not yet arrived. It is the NOW that determines our life." He emphasized that this is why it is so comforting and tranquil to focus on our breath: We become attached to the present, and stop regretting the past or fearing the future.

He then suggested I do Moses's healing prayer with breathing techniques. He said that the great Kabbalists Moses Cordovero and Abraham Abula-fia used mystical breathing techniques. He also said that these breathing techniques reveal that breathing is an art, just as prayer is an art. And if I did the healing prayer of Moses together with proper breathing, I could become an instrument or pure channel through which God's Breath would touch and help heal Jeffrey of his cancerous lesions.

"Remember, Douglas," he concluded, "proper breathing connects you with the Holy Spirit that God breathed into you when you were created." It was as if Rabbi Yaakov turned on a light within me. I intuitively knew at that moment that through proper breathing with the healing prayer, Jeffrey's health would improve dramatically. And it did!

HOW TO: The Healing Prayer of Moses Together with Rabbi Nachman's Teaching on Breathing

1. Sit in in a comfortable chair in a comfortable place, with your back upright. If possible, unbuckle your belt and/or loosen your pants. The person you are praying for sits comfortably next to you.

2. Sit still and focus your awareness on your breathing, be aware of the breathing process. As you inhale through your nostrils, notice the way your abdomen begins to swell and rise. Feel the *Ru'ach* move through your nostrils into your lungs.

3. Trust the Universe — let go and let God. You do this by handing over your breathing to God, by letting your body breathe naturally. Recognize that your breath and God's breath are one breath.

4. When you have done this you are ready to combine the healing prayer with breathing technique. Be aware when this is so.

5. After you have become aware continuously of your breath and God's breath as one, recollect the mantra *Ner Adonai Nishmat Adam, The Light of the Lord is my Soul.* Say this mantra ten times, preferably in Hebrew because of the vibrational power of the Hebrew letters.

   An alternate interpretation of this text is found in Reb Nachman's magnum opus, *Likutei Moharan* I, 60, 3, p. 71b. Reb Nachman, as you may recall, teaches that the Hebrew word *Neshamah*, soul, is related to the Hebrew word *Nishimah*, breath. With this insight, we can re-state the Biblical verse as *The Light of the Lord is my breathing, Ner Adonai Neshimahti.*[4] Say this mantra ten times, either in Hebrew or in English.

6. Concentrate on your love for God, God's love for you, and the love you have for the individual you are praying for. You cannot hold resentment for the person you are praying for, nor can he or she hold resentment for you.

7. Stand up and extend your arms in front of you at eye level, with your palms facing upwards. Breathe in through your nostrils, intuiting silently to a count of six, as you visualize three columns of *Ru'ach*, light, coming down from the heavens — one into each of your hands and one into *Keter* at the crown of your head. Concentrate and visualize the light. As you inhale through your nostrils, your internal dynamic is such that you feel God's *Ru'ach,* breath, co-mingled with the light coming into the palms and fingers of your hands. *Ru'ach* now becomes *Ru'ach HaKodesh.*

8. Turn your hands so that your palms face the person who needs healing. Hold your breath to a count of three.

9. As you exhale through your nostrils, intuiting to the count of six, pour this light onto the person's body. As you do this, feel God's healing light/*Ru'ach HaKodesh* leaving the palms and fingers of your hands and going onto and into the person who needs healing. Be also aware that God's light is continuously entering the middle column through *Keter*, replenishing the light/healing that you are delivering to your friend.

10. As the palms of your hands continue to shine light, light which is being replenished by the middle column of light coming through *Keter,* recite out loud *El Na Rifa Na La* five times and then say once in English: *O God, heal (person's name) now.*

11. Now focus your hands on the specific organ (or other affected body part) you are praying for (instead of the whole body). Next, as you breathe in gently and deeply through your nostrils to a count of six, visualize and feel God's breath/light entering you through the middle column of light. Then hold your breath to a count of three. As you exhale, silently count to six — 1, 2, 3, 4, 5, 6. As you do, visualize and feel God's divine breath/light move from your hands into the organ or limb of the person you are praying for. Then say aloud: *El Na Rifa Na La* five times and *O God, heal _____ now,* one time. After that, passionately, silently, add any prayer you want to offer in your own words while breathing naturally.

12. As always, it is crucial that you know that you are a channel delivering God's healing breath. See this breath as light. I see it as gold/white light. You can see it as any color you want.

13. See the person you are praying for completely healed. Say your own prayers of thanks to God for this healing. We say this with the faith of the Baal Shem Tov: *When we pray we pray as if the prayer has already been answered.*

After doing this healing prayer a number of times, so that you are intimately familiar with it, you don't need to meticulously follow the count 6–3–6. After a while, you will intuitively count. Follow your intuition and don't get bogged down by counting.

The focus of this prayer is on the breath. Rabbi Yaakov was quite clear that the power of the prayer is increased when one identifies one's breath with God's breath, so that we have *Ru'ach HaKodesh.* The action of breathing in and breathing out indicates the continuous Presence of God in our life. The Torah teaches that with each and every breath, we must praise the Lord. We must embrace the Present and know with certainty that the person prayed for is being healed now. That is why we pray knowing our prayer is already answered.

As you become more fluent in Moses's healing prayer with the breath, you can increase the voltage of this prayer by visualizing the co-mingling of *Adonai* אדני and *YHVH* יהוה in every cell of the organ or limb that you want healed, including every cell in the person's body.

NOTES

1. *Sefer Yetzirah,* Chapter 2: *Mishna* 2.
2. *Sefer Yetzirah*, Chapter 2, *Mishna* 3.
3. Observant Jews traditionally say the *Amidah* prayer three times each day — morning, afternoon, and evening. Its purpose is to help us recognize God's sovereignty over all of us. It allows us to thank God for the material and spiritual blessings He bestows upon us, and it encourages us to petition God for the prosperity of ourselves and our loved ones.
4. This teaches that when we breathe correctly and fully, recognizing that His breath is our breath, God's light burns brightly within us and God's soul shines strongly in us.

Rabbi Yaakov Dresher and the Holy Name *Yah*

As I mentioned earlier, I was very touched that Rabbi Yaakov took me under his wing even though I am not an Orthodox Jew. I found his gracious openness to me very inspiring, and I promised to take his knowledge and wisdom very seriously.

He emphasized the importance of accepting that God is everywhere, and seeing God as the Living Breath that fills the universe. He said, "Douglas, before you begin to practice any healing, you must do spiritual exercises, filling yourself up with the Energy or Breath of God every morning." He insisted that I do the traditional Jewish morning prayer service every day. Thanks to him, I can't say often enough that it is crucial to become One with God if you want to practice healing.

I remember he said, "You need *Ru'ach* to do healing. You need to identify your breath with God's Breath. You need to become one with God to the extent that you feel the Presence of God surging through your blood."

"How do I do that?"

"Do you know what the Hebrew expression *Hallelu-Yah* means?"

"Sure. It means 'Praise God.'"

Rabbi Yaakov said, "That's correct. *Hallelu-Yah* means *Praise Yah*. The Hebrew scriptures have many names for the God of the ancient Israelites, including *Elohim, El Shaddai,* and *YHVH*. When the ancient Israelites safely crossed the Red Sea and saw God's great miracle, they sang 'My strength and my song is *Yah*' (Exodus 15:2)."

"Yes," I replied, remembering that *Yah* is an ancient Hebrew name of God. It's a contraction of *YHVH*, and it occurs more than fifty times in the Hebrew scriptures. King David used this Name often in his Psalms, and it is the first divine name used by the author of *Sefer Yetzirah,* the oldest Kabbalistic text.

In his mystical commentaries to the Torah, Isaac Luria maintains that there is an angel who guards and safely delivers all our prayers from earth to heaven. This angel elevates our prayers with the power of *Yah.* Rabbi Yaakov taught me that to pray effectively, I would need to learn from the angels and use the divine name *Yah* in my meditative prayers.

Rabbi Yaakov also instructed me in how we can identify God's breath with our own breath by means of special breathing meditations with God's name, *Yah.* He pointed out that we learn from the Babylonian Talmud (*Menachot* 29) that this physical world we live in was created by the Hebrew letter *Hey* and the world of heaven was created by the Hebrew letter *Yod.* When we put these two letters, or divine energies, together, they form the divine name *Yah.* And when we do meditations on *Yah,* together with special breathing techniques, great healings can ensue.

יָהּ

In the name *Yah,* the letter *Yod* is identified with the masculine and the letter *Hey* is identified with the feminine. The *Yod* is associated with the *Sefira* of *Chochma,* Wisdom, while *Hey* represents the *Sefira* of *Bina,* Understanding. The apex of the *Yod* represents the *Sefira* of *Keter.* In *gematria,* the *Yod* has the numerical value of ten, while *Hey* has the numerical value of five. So this ancient name of *Yah* has the numerical value of fifteen.

Rabbi Yaakov said often, "Know that *Yah* is all around you. When you identify with *Yah,* when you and *Yah* become one, you will be filled up with the breath of God. Your energy will vibrate at a very healthy level and you will be in a position to become a channel for God's healing to take place." He taught me how to achieve this unified state in which my breath and God's breath are one.

If you do the meditations in this chapter in your home, remember to do them in a place that you dedicate consistently to your meditative activity. It can be your living room or your dining room or your bedroom. It doesn't matter what room. What is important is that you use the same room every time so that you create a holy space, with holy energy. You create what the ancient mystics called a *mi'at meekdash,* a small sanctuary, as I suggest throughout this book.

I have a room at home where I draw, study, and pray. Whenever I enter it, I feel a great sense of holiness. In our synagogue, we do healing prayers in front of our Ark. Everyone with whom I pray for healing immediately feels the enormous power of God's energy when the Ark is opened. Such is the power of a space dedicated to holy prayer.

HOW TO: Become a Channel of God's Healing Energy Using the Name of God *Yah*

1. Go to your *mi'at meekdash* and sit in a comfortable chair with your back in the upright position, and your feet planted firmly on the floor. Wear comfortable clothing and loosen up your tie or belt.

2. Breathe in deeply and gently through your nostrils and count silently 1, 2, 3, 4, 5, 6, 7, 8, 9, 10: this is the numerical equivalent of *Yod.* As you breathe in, don't try to visualize God's breath coming in through your nostrils; instead, visualize with your *ko'ach dimyon,* imagination, that God's breath or energy is filling your head area.

3. Without holding your breath between inhaling and exhaling, exhale through your nostrils silently, counting 1, 2, 3, 4, 5: this is the numerical equivalent of *Hey.* The exhaling should take half as long as the inhaling. As you breathe out, don't try to visualize God's breath leaving your nostrils; instead visualize God's breath or energy flowing from your head into your heart and through your heart into the world.

4. Repeat this cycle four times, for a total of five times for the entire meditation. When you inhale or exhale, maintain the internal dynamic that you are breathing in the Life Force of God, and that your breath and His breath are becoming One. Recognize within the depths of your soul that you are becoming one with the Holy Spirit, *Ru'ach HaKodesh.* When we breathe in God's *Ru'ach* with *kavvanah,* we create *Ru'ach HaKodesh;* that is, we become One with the Holy Spirit.

After Rabbi Yaakov practiced this ancient Kabbalistic breathing meditation with me several times, he proceeded to share a more advanced form of it. He maintained that the advanced healing practitioner who wants to fill him- or herself up with the breath of God does not focus on the counting of one through ten. Rather, an experienced practitioner, after many weeks of doing the above meditation, is able to *intuit* the count of ten and the count of five. In addition, the advanced practitioner should be aware of the presence of *Yod* and *Hey* as described in the "increased voltage" version below.

HOW TO: Become a Channel of God's Healing Energy Using the Name of God *Yah*, with Increased Voltage

1. Go to your *mi'at meekdash* and sit in a comfortable chair with your back upright and your feet planted firmly on the floor. Wear comfortable clothing and loosen your tie or belt.

2. Breathe in deeply and gently through your nostrils. As you breathe in, intuit to the count of 1, 2, 3, 4, 5, 6, 7, 8, 9, 10, and be aware of and visualize the letter *Yod* י in your head. Don't try to visualize God's breath coming in through your nostrils; instead, see with your *ko'ach dimyon,* imagination, that God's breath or energy is filling your head area. As you inhale the breath of God and intuit the count of ten while being aware of *Yod* י in your head, hear the sound *ya.*

3. Without holding your breath between inhaling and exhaling, exhale through your nostrils and use your intuition to feel the silent count of 1, 2, 3, 4, 5. The exhaling should take half as long as the inhaling. As you exhale intuiting the count, be aware of and visualize the letter *Hey* ה in your heart. Your vision should not be that God's breath is leaving your nostrils but, rather, that God's breath or energy is flowing from your head into your heart and through your heart into the world. As you intuit the five count and visualize God's breath or energy flowing from your head to your heart into the world, be aware of the Hebrew letter *Hey* ה in your heart, silently vocalize the sound *hhhhh.*

4. When you inhale or exhale, maintain the internal dynamic that you are breathing in the Life Force of God, and that your breath and His

breath are becoming One. Recognize within the depths of your soul that you are becoming one with the Holy Spirit, *Ru'ach HaKodesh.*

5. What you are doing in this meditation is unifying the two letters *Yod Hey* יה and the two sounds — *ya hhhhh* — that make up the name of God and the breath of God. In this way, your breath and God's breath become One and God's *Ru'ach,* through you, becomes *Ru'ach HaKodesh.* You are allowing for the Divine Presence to be within you. When you do either of these spiritual techniques in the morning, you allow yourself to be filled with the Holy Spirit. This greatly increases your ability to be an instrument of God that brings healing to others. You are then in a position to deliver God's healing to another through your prayers.

6. Repeat the meditation four times, for a total of five cycles.

Rabbi Yaakov shared yet another meditative technique based on God's holy name of *Yah* with me. He taught that when you feel that the flow of God's breath within you is vibrating at a low level, and that you need to fill yourself up with a free flow of high vibrational energy, then it is good to stand with your feet close together as if you are standing for the *Amidah*[1] prayer. Interlock the fingers and thumbs of both hands together in front of you with your arms extended fully downward. This locks in the circuit and helps prevent the escape of God's energy. In this position, do rhythmic breathing as described below. I do this meditative exercise with others to increase a free flow of high vibrational energy.

HOW TO: Increase God's Vibrational Energy within You

In this meditation, our numerical count is 6–3–6, rather than 10–5.

1. Go to your *mi'at meekdash* and stand with your chest, neck, and head in a straight line. Wear comfortable clothing and loosen your tie or belt. Extend your arms downward and interlock the fingers and thumbs of both hands together in front of you.

2. Inhale the breath of God gently and deeply through your nostrils, silently counting 1, 2, 3, 4, 5, 6. Hold your breath to the count of 1, 2, 3, and then exhale through your nostrils, counting 1 to 6 again.

3. Maintain the internal dynamic that God's breath becomes One with

yours as you breathe. You are transforming God's *Ru'ach* into *Ru'ach HaKodesh,* or the Holy Spirit within you.

4. As you breathe in through your nostrils, don't visualize that God's breath is coming in through your nostrils, but rather see God's breath filling your head area. Your breath and God's breath are becoming One. God's Holy Spirit or *Ru'ach HaKodesh* is being created within you. As you breathe out through your nostrils, don't visualize God's Holy Spirit leaving your nostrils, but see it flowing from your head into your heart, *and staying in your heart.* Remember, the circuit is closed by the clasping of your fingers. You are becoming more and more filled up with the powerful Presence of God.

5. Do this rhythmic breathing a total of five times, not allowing for the escape of God's energy. This powerfully recharges the Presence of God within you.

Practice these three meditative techniques regularly. We need to practice the Divine Presence as much as we practice for an instrument or a sport. It takes a while to become fluent in these meditations. Don't be discouraged, because when you do master them, the rewards are enormous. You are making yourself into a channel for the Living God, allowing His/Her breath to become one with yours. This is truly a Divine gift.

NOTES

1. The Hebrew word *Amidah* means *standing*, and we are obligated to stand while reciting this prayer. See also note 3, Chapter 12, page 180.

The Healing Prayer of Jeremiah

I N 586 BCE, the ancient Israelites experienced their greatest catastrophe up to that time — the horrific destruction of the great Temple in Jerusalem, a wonder of the ancient world. It was here that they had been able to manifest in a standing building what the traveling Mosaic Tabernacle had been in the wilderness. During that time, the *Mishkan,* or Tabernacle, served as a portal through which our Hebrew ancestors, by means of animal sacrifices and priestly devotion to Torah, could reach God.

The Temple was built under the reign of Solomon because he was a king of peace and the Lord wanted the Temple to be built with hands that were not bloodstained. It was the focal point of our faith, where the priests and Levites and Israelites came together regularly in worship.

But then came Babylonian armies, under the ruthless power of Nebuchadnezzar. After many, many months of battle, the Temple was laid bare and the Israelites were sent into exile in Babylon. The Temple and the king's palace in Jerusalem were burned to the ground.

With no more Temple, what would the Israelites do? They had built their faith around the sacrificial cult practiced there, which was modeled after the desert Tabernacle described in Exodus. How could they continue with their faith, as the Babylonian exile was completely changing the character of their religious practice? A new form of worship had to be established. And it was: The sacrifice of animals was replaced by sacrifice of the lips — prayer.

The prophet Jeremiah lived in this period of much destruction. He saw the Babylonians destroy Nineveh during the Israelite King Josiah's historic seventh-century Israelite reformation. He also saw Josiah's death in the war against the Egyptians. He was alive during the destruction of the great Temple and survived the catastrophe of Jerusalem's conquest and destruction. During Jeremiah's life, the faith of ancient Israel changed from the Hebrew religion to the religion of Judaism, seeds of which developed in Babylon.

After the Persian monarch Cyrus conquered Babylon in 539 BCE, he allowed the Jewish community of Babylon to return to Israel if they so desired. Many of the returning exiles understood that a new religious polity had to be established: This time the religious community would have prayer as a foundation rather than the sacrificial cult.

The spiritual leaders of that persuasion faced a formidable task in creating this new polity. Remembering the prayers of Abraham and Sarah, Rebecca and Isaac and Jacob, Leah and Rachel, even the prayers of Moses, they did all they could to institute the gift of prayer. Even as animal sacrifice resumed with the building of the Second Temple, new communities of prayer dotted the land of ancient Israel as well. As construction of the Second Temple was beginning, our religion already was changing radically. The priestly class was now joined by a scholarly class, called rabbis. These rabbis recognized that oral prayer could have the same spiritual force as sacrifice.

One spiritual community of 120 men became known as the Men of the Great Assembly. It consisted of scholars and rabbis and priests who came together in ways that were very influential in transforming the Hebrew faith into a new Jewish religion. The greatest prayer these men created in the early years of the Second Temple was the prayer of the *Shemoneh Esrai,* the prayer of the Eighteen Blessings.

Of all the prayers of that time, the *Shemoneh Esrai* was, and still is, the most important. *Shemoneh Esrei* means eighteen. It contains eighteen different blessings — some that recognize God's sovereignty, some that express gratitude, some that invoke God for blessings of prosperity, protection of the land of Israel, and peace. Initially, there were eighteen blessings. Later, one additional blessing was added, so that now we pray nineteen blessings, though we didn't change the name of the prayer.

This prayer is so important that observant Jews say it three times each day. It is so important that the Men of the Great Assembly gave the *Shemoneh Esrei* another name, *HaTefilah — The* Prayer — indicating that this prayer stands head and shoulders above all other prayers.

The Eighth Blessing: The Jeremiah Prayer of Healing

The eighth blessing of the *Shemoneh Esrei* is based on two important prayers in Hebrew scripture. One is in Jeremiah 17:14, where Jeremiah calls out to God, "Heal me, O Lord, and let me be healed. Save me and let me be saved. For You are my glory."[1]

The other is in Exodus 15:26, "He [God] said, if you will heed the Lord your God diligently, doing what is upright in His sight, giving ear to His commandments and keeping all His laws, then I will not bring upon you any of the diseases . . ."

רְפָאֵנוּ יהוה וְנֵרָפֵא, הוֹשִׁיעֵנוּ וְנִוָּשֵׁעָה כִּי תְהִלָּתֵנוּ אָתָּה. וְהַעֲלֵה רְפוּאָה שְׁלֵמָה לְכָל־מַכּוֹתֵינוּ.

כִּי אֵל מֶלֶךְ רוֹפֵא נֶאֱמָן וְרַחֲמָן אָתָּה. בָּרוּךְ אַתָּה יהוה רוֹפֵא חוֹלֵי עַמּוֹ יִשְׂרָאֵל.

Refa'einu Adonai v'neirafeh hoshi'einu v'nivashe'ah ki t'hilateinu atah v'ha'aleh refuah shleimah l'chol makoteinu ki el melech rofeh v'ne'eman v'rachaman atah. Baruch atah Adonai rofeh cholim.

Heal us, Lord, and we shall be healed. Save us and we shall be saved, for You are our praise. Bring complete recovery for all our ailments, for You, God, King, are a faithful and compassionate Healer. Blessed are You, Lord, YHVH, Healer of the sick.[2]

Even though this prayer or blessing is based on the words of God through Moses and Jeremiah, our tradition calls this "Jeremiah's prayer of healing." When I pray for healing with people in my community, I use this prayer together with mystical *kavvanot* or meditative intentions more often than most other prayers.

I have known this prayer since I was a child, and remember swaying back and forth with my grandfathers in the synagogue when we recited it during the weekday services. I remember praying this blessing before I was introduced to healing prayer. When my *zaidie* was very sick, my *bubbe* [grandmother] brought me to his hospital bed at Jewish General Hospital in Montreal, and *Bubbe* and I and *Zaidie's* brother Benjamin prayed this prayer fervently. I also pray this prayer regularly when I recite the *Shemoneh Esrei,* whether I am alone or in a *minyan,* a worship service of at least ten Jews aged thirteen or more.

One afternoon a number of years ago, I was visiting with Rabbi Yaakov, and he asked me, "Douglas, do you know why the eighth blessing of the *Shemoneh* Esrei from Jeremiah and the Men of the Great Assembly and the verse from Exodus from *Moishe Rabbenu* are so important for healing?"

"Because Jeremiah said these words and the Men of the Great Assembly created the eighth blessing from these words, and from the verse that God gave Moses," I replied.

"No, Douglas, think Kabbalah. What do you *receive*? When you look at the eighth blessing of the *Shemoneh Esrei* and the text in Exodus, what do you *receive*?"

"I receive that they are both about healing."

"Douglas, look carefully at the two texts. Show me some similarity that you *receive* from the two verses."

"I remember now. Each Hebrew verse has twenty-seven Hebrew words and both Hebrew texts are about healing. Both Hebrew texts also recognize that *Hashem* is the healer."

"Good. How many letters in the Hebrew alphabet?"

"Twenty-two."

"No. There are twenty-seven. Remember, there are twenty-two regular letters of the *alef bet,* from *alef* to *tav,* but then there are an additional five final letters." (These are special forms of five of the letters when they appear as the final letter in a word.)

"Look at the mystery. Look at the mysticism. Look at the Kabbalah of all this. Douglas, herein lies a great secret of healing. The twenty-seven words in the eighth blessing of *Refa'einu* correspond exactly to the twenty-seven letters used to compose the Torah. Also, remember a Hebrew letter is not only a Hebrew letter. The letters manifest the interactions of the *Sefirot.* The Hebrew letters are filled with divine energy. They contain within them the potential powers of the universe.

"We need to know," he continued, "that twenty-two unique energies were created by the interaction of the *Sefirot* among themselves. These energies are the spiritual source of the letters of the Hebrew alphabet.

There are also five other energies which take the shape of the five final Hebrew letters. These two texts that describe *Hashem* as the Great Healer are filled with divinity and divine energy. Every time you repeat either of them, especially the *Refa'einu* verse, you are bringing great healing to the person you are praying for. You become truly an instrument of *Hashem's* amazing healing power.

"Listen, Douglas," he finished on this theme, "you know that the Men of the Great Assembly who formulated the healing prayer *Refa'einu* and all the other *Amidah* blessings created these blessings with enormous precision, with careful regard to the exact number of letters and words. They knew that each letter is a form of energy. And you know that when you put certain letters in a certain sequence, you create an enormous atomic power. That's why it is crucial to pray those words exactly as they were written and created. We cannot change the words or add or subtract words of our own choosing."

Several years ago, some of the women studying with me to become rabbis wanted to change the first blessing of the *Amidah*. They wanted to add in the Hebrew text the names of the matriarchs to those of the patriarchs. I shared with them exactly what Rabbi Yaakov shared with me, that we can't add new Hebrew words or letters to the original sequence of letters or words. These ancient rabbis understood the atomic power in the sequence of the letters as they exist in all nineteen blessings. I did add the names of the matriarchs into the English translation of our prayers, though, because they were as divinely inspired as our patriarchs, and contributed an equal amount to the greatness of our faith.

But the Great Secret, the great Kabbalistic secret of healing in this healing blessing, *Refa'einu*, is that each word, in the way it is written, is filled with enormous healing atomic power. That's why I use it so often. And when I say it in Hebrew, I truly feel each letter of each word delivering healing energy to the person I am praying for.

Rabbi Yaakov also reminded me of another mystical healing text with twenty-seven Hebrew letters:

כִּי־חַיִּים הֵם לְמֹצְאֵיהֶם וּלְכָל־בְּשָׂרוֹ מַרְפֵּא

"They are life to him who finds them. Healing for his whole body" (Proverbs 4:22).3 The verse tells us that the Hebrew letters are life and healing for all who embrace them.

Rabbi Yaakov shared another insight of Kabbalistic healing, referring back to the Kabbalistic Law of Correspondence (first mentioned in Chapter 2). What is true for one aspect of reality is equally true for another aspect of reality: "As above, so below; as below, so above." The blessing of *Refa'einu* was created with twenty-seven words. He pointed out that these words correspond to the twenty-seven letters with which the Torah was written, each of which is a conduit of unique energy.

He said that when a person is ill, whether it be his liver or heart or skin or whatever, that person is not receiving fully all twenty-seven conduits of energy that are necessary for good health. Within the Kabbalistic model of healing, the source of illness and disease is due to damage caused in one or more of these twenty-seven energy conduits. To remedy this, even if we don't know which energy source is lacking, we need to recite the *Refa'einu* prayer, because it contains within it the energies of all twenty-seven Hebrew letters with which God sustains us and creates and heals at all times.

Healing Secret

The Kabbalistic Law of Correspondence teaches that there is an energetic correlation or correspondence between the twenty-seven-word prayer of Jeremiah's *Refa'einu* prayer and the number of letters in the Hebrew alphabet. We recite this twenty-seven-word prayer to do *tikkun* for the harm caused to any of the twenty-seven conduits of sustenance, and to further draw renewed sustenance and health to the sick person.

Joining Inner and Outer Light

When we recite the *Refa'einu* prayer, we are engaging a divine technology that brings the power of the twenty-seven energy forces into the person we are praying for. In so doing, we are making *tikkun* for harm caused to any of the twenty-seven conduits of sustenance. Understanding this internal dynamic puts you in *Mohin de Gadlut,* the Greater Mind. Only when you embrace and participate in the Greater Mind can healing take place.

Your state of mind when you do healing prayer for another person is crucially important. To create wellness in the lives of the people we pray for, we have to be God-like ourselves. We have to know without a doubt that we are connected to the Light, that we are filled with God from head to toe, and that we are sharing the Divine Presence with the person we are praying for.

It is good to recall here the importance of the Feminine Presence of God in healing. Remember that every healing prayer you do — for yourself or for another person — is much more powerful when you pray not only for yourself or your buddy, but also for the *Shechina*, who is in each of us with this disease. When we pray for the *Shechina* within all who have this disease, we identify the innermost divine spark within ourselves, and within the person we are praying for, with the all-encompassing Divine Essence. This is a key secret of Kabbalistic holographic healing, in which everything is within everything and is reflected in everything. When I identify that I am in everything, and everything is in me, including the *Shechina*, there is healing.

When we are doing healing, especially with the *Refa'einu* prayer, we need to recognize that the twenty-two plus five energy forces are the building blocks of the Reality which is the Tree of Life, in which everything exists in perfection. We are bringing these twenty-seven perfect energy forces into the Tree of Knowledge reality in the world in which we live. With the twenty-seven energy forces of the *Refa'einu* prayer, we are truly creating healing. This is the spiritual technology for healing that God has placed in our hands with the *Refa'einu* prayer of the great prophet Jeremiah. What a Kabbalistic secret of healing!

We see again and again that prayer is not, or should not be, based on a series of supplications: The function of prayer is to identify our inner light with the outer light. We can do this by identifying *Adonai* אדני with *YHVH* יהוה. That is, by aligning the spark of divinity within us with the light of the Transcendent.

When I pray, I frequently combine the healing prayer of Jeremiah with the insights of Rabbi Nachman concerning breath. Jeremiah's prayer then functions in a rhythmic fashion. We breathe in to receive the breath of

God. When that happens, God's *Ru'ach,* His breath, mingles with our breath, and we have within us *Ru'ach HaKodesh,* which we can use to bring healing to the person we are praying for.

Lurianic Kabbalah teaches that God creates the universe each moment by breathing Himself into Himself, and then breathing out this light force made up of the Hebrew letters. The presence of divinity in each cell is what allows for the rhythmic behavior of each cell, since it is the nature of God to constantly breathe in and breathe out. When cells contract, it's as if they are breathing out. When cells expand, it's as if they are breathing in. Kabbalah recognizes that all illness begins at the cellular level, and explains it by the breakdown of this rhythmic behavior of the cells.

Everything in this universe, without exception, has to function in a rhythmic fashion to sustain itself. I call this the Energy of the Rhythmic Miracle. The alignment and balance of this energy leads to physical health. The imbalance of this energy and the breakdown of this rhythmic behavior in the universe leads to disease, illness, and death.

HOW TO: Jeremiah's Prayer Combined with Rabbi Nachman's Prayer

1. You and the person you are praying for should sit facing each other in your *mi'at meekdash.* Before you begin this prayer, recollect prayers that you did in the morning that brought you closer to God.

2. Be conscious of your breathing in and out as you inhale and exhale, gently but deeply, several times.

3. Stand up, and recognize that *Hashem* not only is all around you but also within you. Be mindful that the intention of this prayer is to align the spark of divinity within you with the light force of *Hashem* that is above you and surrounds you.

4. Extend your left arm to about eye level with the left palm and fingers facing upward to the heavens. Extend your right arm so that your right palm and fingers face the person you are praying for.

5. First, focus your attention in your left arm and hand, recognizing for about one minute that you are bringing *Hashem's Ru'ach* into your left hand. Then focus attention in your right arm and hand, with your palm facing the organ you are healing. Recognize that you are delivering *Ru'ach HaKodesh* or healing through the right hand.

6. As you breathe in gently but deeply through your nostrils, visualize

God's *Ru'ach* as a gold/white light coming down through the heavens into your left hand.

7. As you breathe in deeply but gently through your nostrils, feel God's *Ru'ach* travel from the palm of the left hand, up the left arm, across your chest, down your right arm, into the palm of your right hand. This spiritual activity of merging your *Ru'ach* with God's transforms *Ru'ach* into *Ru'ach HaKodesh,* Sacred Breath or Sacred Healing.

8. As you exhale through your nostrils, visualize the *Ru'ach HaKodesh* as a goldish-white light leaving your right hand and entering your friend's affected organ or area. Gently move this light with your right arm rotating counterclockwise all over the affected organ/area.

9. Now recite the Jeremiah prayer:

> *Refa'einu Adonai v'neirafeh hoshi'einu v'nivashe'ah ki t'hilateinu atah v'ha'aleh refuah shleimah l'chol makoteinu ki el melech rofeh v'ne'eman v'rachaman atah. Baruch atah Adonai rofeh cholim.*
>
> *Heal us, Lord, and we shall be healed. Save us and we shall be saved, for You are our praise. Bring complete recovery for all our ailments, for You, God, King, are a faithful and compassionate Healer. Blessed are You, Lord, YHVH, Healer of the sick.*

10. After you say the Jeremiah prayer, add your own words of prayer to God, but remember, it is not a matter of pleading. It is a matter of identifying the spark of God within you with the Transcendent *Hashem.*

11. See your friend, the person you're praying for, completely well, and offer thanks to God for healing her or him. Remember to pray as if your prayer is already answered. We always need to pray in the Greater Mind.

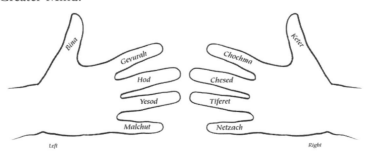

Sometimes we feel that we want to tweak or change our prayer mildly. Do it, follow your intuition. This is God speaking to you. But remember, prayer is not magic. Prayer is our connection to God. It takes time, love, perseverance, and faith. Whenever you do this prayer, or any prayer, it is crucial that you feel love for the person you are praying for and for *Hashem*.

One powerful way of modifying the prayer with *kavvanah* is to mentally identify the five *Sefirot* on the left hand every time you bring in *Hashem's Ru'ach* through breathing in, and then identify the five *Sefirot* on the right hand as you exhale the *Ru'ach HaKodesh* with the right hand.

NOTES

1. JPS (Jewish Publication Society) Hebrew/English Tanakh, 1999.
2. My translation and transliteration vary slightly from the original Hebrew, but I have found my transliteration and translation to be very efficacious in their healing power.
3. JPS (Jewish Publication Society) Hebrew/English Tanakh, 1999.

15

The Healing Prayer of Aaron

I was very young when my father's father Rabbi Haskell Goldhamer passed away. My father told me that his dad was named after Ezekiel, the dreamer prophet. Ezekiel's visions are well-known and studied by all Kabbalists.

I was almost eight years old when *Zaidie* Haskell passed away, and I remember the moment as clearly as if it happened yesterday. It was a Sunday morning in April. The Montreal snow was almost gone. My dad was giving me a piggyback ride when the phone rang. The caller told my father that his papa, my *zaidie*, had died. In one moment, the joy of our household was gone.

I didn't know my father's father well. This doesn't mean I didn't visit him often. In fact, I did. I didn't know him well because I couldn't speak Yiddish or German, and he couldn't speak English or French. We did find common ground, though, in the little Hebrew I knew at that time.

Without a doubt, I was his precious *Dovid* (my Hebrew name). He always looked forward to my visits, and he always bestowed empty cigar boxes upon me. Sometimes they were filled with pencils. He liked to watch me study the Hebrew letters, and the better I did, the more pencils I received. He blessed me each time I visited him. I can't remember his words or even my thoughts, but I will never forget how his eyes looked deeply into mine as he blessed me.

My *zadie* had been a rabbi in Germany. When he came to Montreal, he held the position of Rebbe in a *shteiblich,* a small neighborhood synagogue. He was ninety-seven when he died.

Rabbi Chaim of Volozhin, the great nineteenth-century Vilna Kabbalist and author of *Nefesh HaChayim,* teaches that a true blessing reaches into a person's soul, touches his or her life's purpose, and brings it into this world. A true blessing finds the hidden truth of a person and prays for its realization here. Many years later, I learned that the blessing my *zaidie* offered me each time we met was the ancient priestly blessing with which Aaron blessed the Israelites:

יְבָרֶכְךָ יְהֹוָה וְיִשְׁמְרֶךָ:

יָאֵר יְהֹוָה פָּנָיו אֵלֶיךָ וִיחֻנֶּךָּ:

יִשָּׂא יְהֹוָה פָּנָיו אֵלֶיךָ וְיָשֵׂם לְךָ שָׁלוֹם:

Y'varekhi'khah YHVH v'yishm'rekhah,
Ya'er YHVH panav eilekhah vi'chunekah.
Yisah YHVH panav eilekhah v'yasem lekhah shalom.

May YHVH bless you and keep you.
May YHVH let His face shine upon you and be gracious to you.
May YHVH lift up His spirit upon you and grant you peace.

This blessing is very well known. In addition to hearing it in our synagogue many time, I've also heard it recited in Catholic and Protestant churches. What makes it genuinely remarkable for me, though, is that my grandfather truly healed my soul when he recited this ancient blessing. He healed my soul in that he knew what my future destiny would be, and he brought it into reality. When I was studying to become a rabbi, my father said to me, "This is what your *Zaidie* Haskell really wanted for you."

In my high school years, I studied Talmud regularly in Montreal with Rabbi Lapkofsky. He was a gentle man with a white goatee, and he visited my home every Sunday morning. He continued to unfold the mysteries of the priestly blessing by teaching me its relationship with healing. In our Orthodox synagogue, the priestly blessing was said by the priest as he faced the congregation.[1]

Rabbi Lapkofsky showed me the passage from the Talmud that shows the relationship between this blessing and healing. As the priest recites this blessing before the congregation on holy days, including Passover, Shavuot, and Yom Kippur, the worshippers ask God to heal them as He healed Hezekiah from his "sickness" (Isaiah 38:1–5), Miriam from her leprosy (Numbers 12:10–15), or the waters of Jericho through Elisha (2 Kings 2:19–22), and other instances of miraculous healing.

Peeking through the Window

My grandfather, being both a rabbi and *Cohen,* a Jewish priest, blessed me in the same way he blessed his little Montreal congregation. He used the blessing from Numbers and its Talmudic correlate, found in Tractate *Berakot* 55b. I will always remember how he would extend both his arms with his fingers arranged with the thumbs and index fingers of each hand touching the other, creating a triangle space between the two hands. Before forming the triangle the first two fingers on each hand are held together, separated from the other two touching fingers — like Mr. Spock of *Star Trek*, as illustrated below.

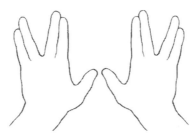

The open spaces between the fingers, according to Judaism, are the "windows" through which God looks. This mystical phenomenon of "peeking through the window" means that the divine Presence peeks through the windows between the fingers. The five spaces refer to the biblical *Song of Songs* or *Shir HaShirim* 2:9, which states that *Hashem* "peeks through the cracks in the wall."[2] *Hashem* watches and protects us always.

My *zadie* used to call this the healing prayer of Aaron, because Aaron, Moses's brother, was the high priest of the Israelites. Aaron was known as a man who dedicated his life more than any other man to the struggle for peace.

The Hebrew word for peace is *shalom.* When we pray for healing, we use a word which is a derivative of *shalom* and say "May you have a *Refuah Shlema*," a *complete* healing. This teaches us that peace and the

completeness of healing are from the same source. Aaron's priestly benediction is not only a prayer for peace, but also an equally powerful prayer
for healing.

God instructed Moses to teach his brother Aaron how to bless the people
of Israel with this prayer. In ancient times, the high priest was not only
the spiritual leader, but also the people's leading physician. The text makes
clear that this specific blessing originates not from the priest, but from God
Himself. The priest is asked to "put My Name upon the people Israel." As
we learn again and again in scripture, God is ultimately the healer. In this
specific blessing, God is using Aaron as His instrument.

This unique blessing has three parts: first, the blessing for material
healing goods; second, the blessing for intellectual healing pursuits; and
third, the blessing for mental, physical, and spiritual healing. My *zaidie*
loved Aaron's blessing.

Remember, *prayer* is your request for yourself, whereas *blessing* is your
request for another. When a person truly blesses another person using
Aaron's priestly blessing, the bestower of blessing gives God great pleasure.

Raising the hands with palms up to God demonstrates a recognition
of the Lord. But when one raises the hands with the palms down, as in
Aaron's blessing, then one acts as a divine instrument receiving and pouring
forth God's divine energy. Sometimes we entreat God to empower us to
do blessings of healing, and sometimes we entreat God to use us as His
divine instrument or vessel. The healer, through intuitive connection with
God, knows what to do when.

Using Aaron's priestly blessing can be very powerful. I place my hands
in the blessing position, palms down, over the recipient's head, allowing
God's divine energy to flow through me, through my hands, onto the
recipient. When Moses raised his hands in healing, he concentrated on his
ten fingers to deliver spiritual energies. Aaron did the same with his priestly
blessing of healing. He would also concentrate on the ten emanations and
the Source of the blessings that flow from the celestial worlds.

When I deliver the Aaronic blessing of healing, I likewise concentrate
on the number ten, focusing on the ten emanations of spiritual energies
originating from the Source of all creation. To concentrate on the number ten is a key secret in Kabbalistic healing, whether you bless using the

left hand/right hand modality of Jeremiah, or the two-handed blessing of Moses, or the priestly blessing of Aaron.

I remember when Jim and Rhonda visited me. Jim is the brother of a member of our synagogue. He had a brain tumor on the right side of his head, near the right temporal lobe. It was non-malignant, but clearly was causing him hardship. He had headaches and, at times, his left hand would shake. He was worried that the tumor would become malignant, even though his doctors advised against such worry. The right side of his head was shaved and he had a bandage on his head. Rhonda, his wife, is an actress who has appeared in commercials and had small parts in movies. She and Jim often go to parties, and he was becoming more and more self-conscious at them, especially after his surgery.

At our first meeting, Jim told me that "they got most of it," but he needed further radiation treatments. "I feel like a freak at my wife's parties," he said. "All these actors are so darn beautiful. Look at me."

I told him I understood, and would try to find the right blessings of healing to do for him. I asked him for a medical description of his situation so that I would better know how to pray over the tumor, and asked if I could speak with his physician. I find it very helpful to speak with people's physicians, as they can really explain the medical condition clearly. I usually ask them, "If prayer were one of your modalities of healing, what would you pray for?" Jim's physician didn't know the cause of his disease, so he simply suggested that we pray for the disappearance of the remaining tumor that the surgery couldn't remove, which was then being treated by radiation.

When I met with Jim and Rhonda a second time, I told them that I approach healing prayer like an internist treats a patient with a certain disease. Suppose the patient is suffering from depression. Doctors often prescribe different medications until one takes hold and works well. I find the experience is similar in prayer. Sometimes a parishioner is more comfortable with one kind of prayer than another. Some may seem too strange to embrace. Others may remind them of prayers they heard in the synagogue when they were young.

A person's chemistry plays a part in how he/she responds to certain medications. I find this to be true spiritually also. Different souls respond differently to the same blessings of healing. It's not that one blessing fits all. After much practice, you will be able to slightly modify a prayer or blessing, so that the person you are offering it to may receive healing. This is another secret of Kabbalistic healing.

I shared with Jim and Rhonda how healing prayer was used in Biblical and Rabbinic Judaism. This seemed to put them at ease, and eliminated any speculation that the healing prayer I was teaching them was New Agey, not rooted in our Jewish scripture.

The first healing prayer we studied was the one Moses used in Miriam's healing, and we did different variations of it for many weeks. We did both Mosaic healing prayers, the one outlined in *This Is for Everyone* and the one in Chapter 11 of this book. But after a few months, the MRI and CT scan showed that the tumor had not disappeared, but actually had grown minimally.

"I knew this wouldn't work," Jim said. "We've never been religious people. I guess our prayers aren't reaching God."

I asked them, "How many children do you have?"

"Four."

"That's a lot of children. Do you love each one of them?"

They laughed. "Of course. They're our children."

"Well, God loves you. You are His children too. We just need to try a different healing meditation. We need to find a perfect fit."

I remembered that both Rhonda and Jim were in a Conservative synagogue in one of the Chicago suburbs. In fact, they met on a synagogue mission to Israel, and I remember Jim telling me back then that he was amazed that this pretty actress could read Hebrew so well. Jim read Hebrew very well and had thought of being a *cantor* when he was younger. He became a chiropractor instead.

Jim also was very proud not only of his Judaism, but of his lineage as a *Cohen*. At one of our meetings, we shared stories about our grandfathers blessing their respective congregations. So I knew that he and Rhonda would relate to and embrace the *Beerkat Cohanim* blessing. I told them I intuitively felt that this healing blessing would have the desired effect and began to teach Rhonda the prayer.

"But she's not a *Cohen* — and she's a woman," Jim said.

"You're right. Isn't it wonderful that your wife could be doing this for you? Isn't it wonderful that we're using the *Beerkat Cohanim* with its healing properties as Aaron envisioned them?"

I taught Rhonda to hold her hands in the priestly position four to six inches over Jim's tumor. As an actress, she saw herself as an ancient priest doing healing, just as in Biblical times.

As Rhonda placed her hands over the remaining tumor, she visualized God's light going through the window spaces of her fingers, penetrating deep into Jim's skull, melting the tumor. The Hebrew text of *Song of Songs* (2:9) speaks of the Light of God as "gazing through the Window, peering through the lattice." It is upon this Biblical text that the rabbis based the finger positions of the hands for this prayer.

"But how do I know this will work?" Rhonda asked.

I reminded her that her hands represent her ability to draw blessings from the celestial world into this physical world. I also reminded her to focus on the number ten, symbolizing the ten *Sefirotic* energies.

I understood that Jim, as a chiropractor and a committed Jew — as is Rhonda — would be interested to know that *Mishna* of Talmud *Ohalot* 1:8 teaches that each hand possesses 30 bones, 14 revealed joints, and 16 concealed joints. These are 30 of the 248 bones that composed the skeleton. These 248 bones parallel the 248 positive commandments. Since each hand contains 30 bones, the two hands contain 60 bones, which correspond to the sixty Hebrew letters of the priestly blessing healing prayer of Aaron.[3]

I shared with Rhonda that, as she places her raised palms over Jim's wound, the light of the sixty letters of this healing blessing emanates from the sixty bones of her hands. Each Hebrew letter contains a different kind of sacred energy, which God continues to use to heal. In the same way, Rhonda was using the Hebrew letters and their holy energies as instruments of God's healing for her husband. She and Jim were inspired. They looked forward to praying with this ancient blessing, and did.

It is now six years since I first met Jim. His tumor is gone. He and his wife are confident, as am I, that it was God, together with their persistent prayer and good medical treatment, that got rid of the tumor.

HOW TO: How to Be an Instrument of Healing Using Aaron's Priestly Blessing of Healing, #1

1. If you intend to pray regularly for someone, whether your spouse or a friend or a family member, you need to have a strong relationship with God to be effective. This means that every morning, in the same place, around the same time, you should thank God for all the gifts — spiritual and physical — that He has given you. Then briefly talk with Him as a person speaks with a close friend. Then hold, with deep aspirational feeling, the thought of the meditative spiritual exercise(s) you want to do.

2. When the time comes to do the exercise with another person, both prayer partners should center yourselves and feel connected to, or filled up, with the Presence of God. This can be done in several ways, using meditations in this book.

3. For Aaron's blessing, place your hands in the priestly position (as described above in "Peeking through the Window") with your palms facing the part of the other person's body that needs healing. Before praying, practice vocalizing the priestly benediction in the original Hebrew letters (remember these sixty Hebrew letters correspond to the sixty bones of the two hands). Sounding the Hebrew words of this healing prayer activates or "turns on" your hands to God's healing energy, by their vibrational power. Also concentrate on the number ten — your ten fingers delivering ten emanations of energies.

4. With your hands in the priestly benediction position over the part of the body that needs healing, recite out loud in Hebrew and in English the first verse of the priestly blessing:

יְבָרֶכְךָ יְהוָה וְיִשְׁמְרֶךָ

Y'varekhi'khah YHVH v'yish'm'rekhah.
May YHVH bless you and keep you.

5. Say the second verse of the priestly blessing in Hebrew and English:

יָאֵר יְהוָה פָּנָיו אֵלֶיךָ וִיחֻנֶּךָּ

Ya'er YHVH panav eilekhah vi'chunekah.
May YHVH let His face shine upon you and be gracious to you.

6. Say the third verse of the priestly blessing:

יִשָּׂא יְהוָה פָּנָיו אֵלֶיךָ וְיָשֵׂם לְךָ שָׁלוֹם

Yisah YHVH panav eilekhah v'yasem lekhah shalom.
May YHVH lift up His spirit upon you and grant you peace.

If you look at English translations of Aaron's blessing in the Book of Numbers, Chapter 6, verses 24–26, you most often see words like "May the Lord bless . . . May the Lord let His face. . . . May the Lord lift up His spirit . . ." This is not accurate. It should say "May *YHVH* . . ." each time. So, with each of these three blessings, you should say "May *YHVH* bless you . . . May *YHVH* let His face shine. . . . May *YHVH* lift up His spirit . . ." And when you say *YHVH*, you should also visualize *YHVH* יהוה on the injured organ in the ten different *Sefirotic* energetic colors.

HOW TO: How to Be an Instrument of Healing Using Aaron's
Priestly Blessing of Healing, #2

1–3. Same as for Aaron's Priestly Blessing of Healing #1 above.

4 a) Breathe in gently through your nostrils, counting silently to six. While breathing in and counting, visualize a beam of gold/white light infused with purple sets of *YHVH* יהוה entering your skull, through *Keter,* and continuing downward until it rests in your heart, which is *Tiferet.*

b) Hold your breath to the count of three (silently) and visualize your heart, *Tiferet* area, filled with this light.

c) As you exhale gently through your nostrils to the silent count of six, visualize God's light moving out of your heart, traveling across your chest, down your arms, and flowing through the windows of your hands, entering your friend's affected area, transforming the tumor cells into healthy cells. Then recite the first verse of the priestly blessing:

יְבָרֶכְךָ יְהוָה וְיִשְׁמְרֶךָ

Y'varekhi'khah YHVH v'yishm'rekhah.
May YHVH bless you and keep you.

5. Repeat steps 4a through 4c, except at the end recite the *second* verse of the priestly blessing:

יָאֵר יְהוָה פָּנָיו אֵלֶיךָ וִיחֻנֶּךָּ

Ya'er YHVH panav eilekhah vi'chunekah.
May YHVH let His face shine upon you and be gracious to you.

6. As above, repeat steps 4a through 4c except this time at the end recite the *third* verse of the priestly blessing:

יִשָּׂא יְהוָה פָּנָיו אֵלֶיךָ וְיָשֵׂם לְךָ שָׁלוֹם

Yisah YHVH panav eilekhah v'yasem lekhah shalom.
May YHVH lift up His spirit upon you and grant you peace.

7. Now visualize the sets of *YHVH* יהוה joining with the *Adonai* אדני, *Alef Dalet Nun Yod*, of each cell in the affected area, so that you visualize the יאהדונהי energy in each cell. Each cell now has balanced male and female energies. You only need to see one cell being transformed, knowing that immediately and instantaneously all the cells are being transformed to יאהדונהי.

8. Visualize your partner completely well, and thank God for healing him or her. Remember the teachings of the Baal Shem Tov and Levi Yitzhak of Berdichev: Pray as if your prayer is already answered.

HOW TO: The Triangle Touch Healing Meditation, Variations Based on the Priestly Healing Benediction of Aaron

In one variation, everything is the same as for Aaron's Priestly Blessing of Healing #1 above, except for one thing to be done each time before you recite the appropriate verse of the priestly blessing. And that is this: As God's light penetrates the tumor or otherwise affected area, visualize the negative energy of the tumor (or other illness) breaking up and escaping through the center of the triangle. I see this as black or gray smoke. Then say the verse as in the previous exercises.

It is also possible to do Aaron's priestly healing blessing by first activating the ten *Sefirot*, lifting up your arms with palms facing upwards, concentrating on the number ten, and remembering the Kabbalistic secrets of the ten fingers we've discussed earlier. Remember that Rabbi Hezekiah teaches that if a person raises his two arms with palms facing upward while in a state of prayer, the ten spiritual powers of the *Sefirot* in us receive blessings from above, and the person doing the blessing can transfer these blessings to the person receiving healing. Rabbi Bachya ben Asher, the great medieval Kabbalist, emphasized that there is great *Sefirotic* power in concentrating on the ten fingers after the arms have been lifted up.

Let's look at a variation based on Rabbi Hezikiah's teachings.

HOW TO: An Alternate Form of Aaron's Healing Prayer, Based on Rabbi Hezekiah's Teachings of the Power of Ten

Preliminary

I usually do this version of Aaron's healing prayer as I sit in front of the Ark with the person I am praying for, who is also seated. I find the healing that results from this blessing to be very strong. So I suggest that, if you want to do this variation with someone, do it somewhere that is very special or holy to that person — a special area of the house, or somewhere that feels sacred to them. If you are praying for someone who is confined to bed, sit facing that person so that either the two of you are seated, or you are seated (at least to begin with) and the other person is lying in bed. Mentally practice reciting to yourself the priestly benediction in the original Hebrew letters while remembering that these sixty Hebrew letters correspond to the sixty bones of the two hands.

Both of you should relax and try to feel the Presence of God.

When you feel the Presence clearly, put your hands in front of you ten inches apart, and identify the five masculine *Sefirot* represented by the five fingers of the right hand and the five feminine *Sefirot* represented by the five fingers of the left hand. As you imagine the *Sefirot* corresponding to the five fingers of each hand, you are polarizing these *Sefirot* and creating strong spiritual tension. This tension is the divine energy within you.

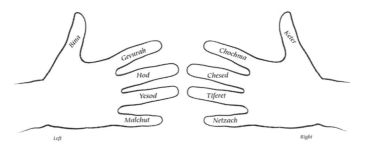

Begin the Healing Prayer

1. Facing the other person, stand with your arms outstretched at shoulder level toward the sky with your palms and fingers facing upwards. Concentrate on the number ten. Concentrate on the fact that your ten fingers represent the ten *Sefirot* and that you are receiving ten golden strings of light, one string in each finger. Also visualize a beam of light coming down from the heavens onto the crown of your head. This beam of infinite light constantly replenishes the ten strings of golden light, as we've discussed in earlier exercises using this modality.

2. Turn your palms facing the person you are praying for, and focus on the area of his or her body that needs healing.

3. The fingers of both of your hands should now be in the "Spock" priestly blessing arrangement facing the affected area: index fingers touch middle fingers, fourth fingers and pinkies touch, hands are separate from each other.

Concentrate on the fact that your ten fingers represent the ten *Sefirot* by silently naming the *Sefira* corresponding with each your ten fingers, and that a beam of gold/white light from the heavens rests on the crown of your head. Breathe in gently and deeply through your nostrils. Know as you do this that your fingers are being replenished with God's divine light through *Keter*. Then, as you exhale, visualize ten golden strings of *Sefirotic* healing light streaming from your fingers and healing the injured organ or limb or area, while you recite the first verse of the priestly blessing:

יְבָרֶכְךָ יְהוָה וְיִשְׁמְרֶךָ

Y'varekhi'khah YHVH v'yish'm'rekhah.
May YHVH bless you and keep you.

4. With your hands in the same position, breathe in deeply and gently and feel God's divine light entering through the crown of your head. As you exhale, again visualize the ten golden beams of light healing the limb or organ while you recite the second verse of the prayer:

יָאֵר יְהוָה פָּנָיו אֵלֶיךָ וִיחֻנֶּךָּ

Ya'er YHVH panav eilekhah vi'chunekah.
May YHVH let His face shine upon you and be gracious to you.

5. Repeat step four, but at the end this time recite the third verse of the prayer:

יִשָּׂא יְהוָה פָּנָיו אֵלֶיךָ וְיָשֵׂם לְךָ שָׁלוֹם

Yisah YHVH panav eilekhah v'yasem lekhah shalom.
May YHVH lift up His spirit upon you and grant you peace.

6. As a result of your focusing on the spiritual force of the ten *Sefirot,* the Hebrew words that you said became filled with mystical healing power. The ancients would say your tongue became circumcised, and you were able to use the mysteries of the Hebrew language. Your healing blessings of Aaron and Hezekiah have had their proper effect. Visualize your prayer partner completely well, and recite: *Hodu l'Adonai kee tov kee l'Olam chasdo, O Give Thanks to the Lord for His healing is forever.*

As you see, there are many versions and many ways of interpreting the Aaronic blessing of healing. Each version, each modality is good. As I say again and again, a key Kabbalistic healing secret is that no single healing prayer fits all. It is up to you, as an instrument of God's healing, to discover and decide which blessing will work best in the person you are praying with.

I do this by first talking with the person I will be praying for. Perhaps I even play air hockey with him. I get a handle on what he or she is like. This helps me decide what prayer I will use. I also try to speak with the person's physician. Then, I pick one of the prayers and try it for a number of weeks. If I see that this prayer connects intuitively with the other person, and that it is helping spiritually and medically, I continue with it. If, after six weeks or two months, I don't see improvement, I try another version of the same prayer, or another prayer altogether.

Don't be afraid to try several versions. When you have become fluent in various modalities, you might even want to combine two of the prayers into one. Through practice and more practice, you will be able to use these prayers as fluently as you drive your car. Don't be afraid. Continue to trust God, and trust that God wants you to do this healing work. Through practice and personal prayer on a regular basis, you will be able to intuit what God wants you to do.

NOTES

1. The Jewish spiritual leader in biblical times was part of the priestly class. The only way one could become a priest was to be male and born of a father who was a priest. It was an inherited position. Nonetheless, the son who inherited the mantle had to do an enormous amount of studying before he could be an active priest. Jewish people today continue to trace their descent through the priestly class. I find it amazing that my grandfather was a priest, my father was a priest, and I, in addition to being a rabbi, am a priest.

2. There are different traditions as to the placement of the hands for the Priestly Blessing. Some *Cohanim* put their two hands together so that they form the Hebrew letter *Shin*, which symbolizes the *Shechina*. My grandfather would first place his hands so that *Hashem* could "peek through the window" and then he would move his hands to create a triangle between the two hands.

3. Although traditional Judaism, including the Mishna and Kabbalistic texts such as *Be'er Mayim Chayim* by Rabbi Chaim of Chernovitz, maintain that the hand has 30 bones, and the body has 248 bones, modern science tells us that the hand is composed of 27 bones and 206 bones comprise the human body by adulthood. I believe that this fact does not negate the close connection between the Priestly Blessing and hands. However, it does show how polite Jim the chiropractor is, since he chose not to contradict me when I shared this information with him.

16

Healing Yourself and Healing Others
Teachings of Rabbi Nachman of Breslov

Much of the healing that I have shared with you in this work so far requires two people — an instrument of God to deliver the healing and an instrument of God to receive the healing. The Talmud maintains, as explained earlier, that it is very difficult to heal oneself, because it is very difficult for a person in great physical or mental pain to be completely in the Greater Mind, free of negative thoughts. That's why healing prayer in *chevruta*-like study is recommended: One member of the prayer team is filled with the Greater Mind through love for God and for the person he or she is praying for, and the other person can draw inspiration and even faith from that prayer partner.

There is one modality of prayer, however, that allows and even encourages the person who is ill to pray for him- or herself. This modality is based on the teachings of Rabbi Nachman of Breslov. Many of Rabbi Nachman's healing teachings are found dispersed throughout his multi-volume work, *Likutei Moharan,* the *Collected Writings of Rabbi Nachman of Breslov.*[1] The thrust of his healing teaching is that sickness is a result of depression. And, turning this upside down, Rabbi Nachman sees that the greatest healer is joy.

When I was first diagnosed with Klippel-Trenaunay syndrome some forty years ago, there was very little that could put me in a state of joy. I was in constant pain. I understood the Talmudic teaching that it is difficult for a very ill person to deliver himself out of the prison of sickness. Yet I was intrigued by Rabbi Nachman's teachings that not only can we pray for ourselves, but joy is the key to wellness.

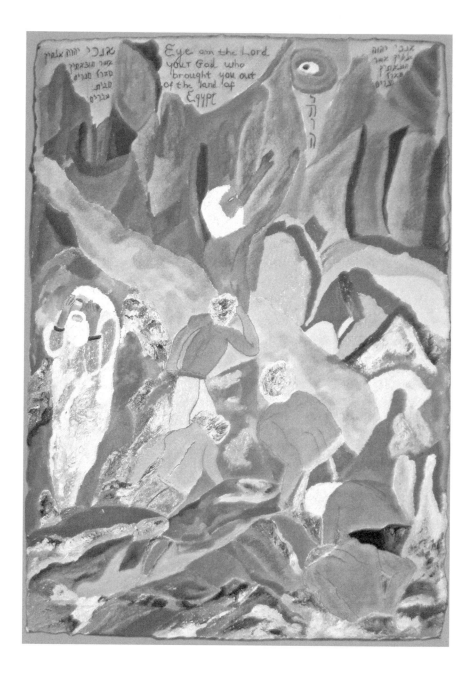

Rabbi Nachman teaches that there is a direct relationship between sickness in the body and sickness in the soul. His teachings are very Kabbalistic, expressing holistic and holographic ideas, especially in his instructions on how to heal ourselves. The great Hasidic teacher Rabbi Dov Baer (1704–1772) paraphrased Rabbi Nachman's teachings as, "A small hole in the body, a big hole in the soul."

Rabbi Nachman taught that healing is only possible when we recognize that God is within every cell of our body. Each of us is a unique expression of God. When we believe that we are separate from God, that we are not filled with God in every cell from head to toe, this false thinking makes a person susceptible to illness. Embracing this false notion is just as dangerous as living without joy. Both are roots of all illness, according to Rabbi Nachman. He believed strongly that spiritual healing leads to physical healing.

He was also a great believer in the Kabbalistic principle of *Spiritual Balance*. An individual should recognize that he or she is a unique manifestation of the Deity, with emphasis on *unique* and on *Deity*. There must always be a spiritual balance between the individual's belief in her- or himself and the belief that s/he is completely filled in every cell with the Presence of God.

Rabbi Nachman embraced the concept that each of us has the power, through words, to speak to a limb or an organ of our body that is ill or damaged or hurt. He had conviction that if we have heart disease, or liver disease, or malfunctioning intestines or kidneys, or a broken arm, or tumors in our abdomen or head, or other illness in another part of the body, we need to speak to these affected parts and encourage them to heal themselves.

Rabbi Nachman taught that we should regularly go to a secluded place and meditate and talk with God. He was very much influenced in this by Rabbi Chaim Vital, who called this kind of dialogue with God *hitbodidut*.[2] If your liver, for example, is diseased, Rabbi Nachman would suggest that during this quiet time of *hitbodidut* meditation with God, you should ask God to heal your liver. Then he would have you talk directly to your liver. He would want you to talk to the soul of the liver.

How is that possible? Because our soul exists everywhere, in every cell, throughout the body. Soul and body are one. *Hitbodidut* translates into

English as"enclothement" and involves associating specific spiritual powers with limbs and organs of the body. It demonstrates the Kabbalistic concept of vesting a higher order of reality in a lower one. We see the higher reality, the soul or a power of the soul, "enclothed" by and expressing itself through the medium of a lower reality, a physical vessel such as a limb or organ of the body.

In this instance, the lower reality is the liver, and the higher reality is the soul. Recognizing the holographic nature of every cell of the body, and the Kabbalistic principle that everything is in everything, Rabbi Nachman naturally recognized that God set up Reality as a complex superstructure with many sublevels or systems within systems. Every cell of our liver is a composite of the ten *Sefirot*.

Anthropomorphically speaking, the three higher *Sefirot*, *Keter, Chochma*, and *Bina*, represent the *brains* or *soul* of the *Sefirotic* Tree, while the seven lower *Sefirot* are the *body* of the Tree. Rabbi Nachman's spiritual teachings on healing require that the individual with liver disease speak to the soul of the liver, and then speak to the soul of each liver cell, since holographically and Kabbalistically, each liver cell — as a living expression of this Tree — has a soul.

I find Rabbi Nachman's teachings valuable and efficacious when applied on a regular basis, several times a day. In the past few years, I have prayed with many people with liver diseases such as hepatitis, liver cancer, secondary cancer in the liver, or cirrhosis of the liver. We have seen great success with the following prayer, which is based on the teachings of Rabbi Nachman of Breslov, Rabbi Chaim Vital, and Lurianic Kabbalah.

HOW TO: Healing Cell Meditation, Based on the Prayers of Rabbi Nachman of Breslov

1. Wearing relaxed clothing, go to your *mi'at meekdash*. Sit in a comfortable chair or, if sitting is too difficult, lie down.
2. Breathe in and out naturally.
3. Gently, be conscious of your breathing and aware that God is with you and within you.
4. Speak with your liver, or other affected organ, as Rabbi Nachman of

Breslov teaches. Say, "I love you, my liver (or other affected organ), I love you very much. You have been with me all these years, keeping me strong, healthy, and alive. I love you, the soul of my liver. And I ask you, the soul of my liver, to energize my liver body. I also ask you, the soul of each cell of my liver, to inspire each cell to work well and to take care of itself, and to repair itself, and to love itself. I ask you, the soul of each liver cell, to love the cell in which you reside. I love each soul of each liver cell. You are wonderful. Please inspire each cell to repair itself. I love you, each liver cell. Strong, well, and healthy liver cells . . . healthy cells . . . (say eight times). I see each liver cell very healthy. Healthy liver cells, healthy liver cells. I see a healthy and wonderful liver. You are a healthy and wonderful liver. I love you my liver (say ten times). Thank you, the soul of my liver for bringing healing. Thank you the soul of each liver cell for bringing healthy repair and healing. Thank you God for giving me a healthy liver. I love you my liver. I love you my God."

This prayer can be done with any organ or limb or affected part — such as your lungs or heart or kidneys or legs or arms — by substituting the name of the appropriate organ or limb and the appropriate organ or limb cells. It also can be used with increased voltage by correcting the spiritual imbalance of cells filled only with feminine divine energies, as outlined below.

HOW TO: Healing Cell Meditation of Rabbi Nachman of Breslov, with Increased Voltage

1–3. Same as 1–3 above.

4. Similar to 4 above, except here say only this much: *I love you, my liver (or other affected organ). I love you very much. You have been with me all these years, keeping me strong, healthy and alive. I love you, the soul of my liver. And I ask you, the soul of my liver, to energize my liver body.*

5. Visualize a beam of light from the heavens coming through the roof, onto the *Keter* of your head. This beam of light is the Transcendent Male aspect of God, and is filled with numerous sets of *YHVH* יהוה. (I often visualize these characters as purple.) As you

breathe in through your nostrils, visualize these sets of *YHVH* יהוה divine masculine energies entering every cell of your body, including your liver cells.

6. Now say: *I ask you, the souls of each cell of my liver to inspire each cell to work well and to take care of itself, to repair itself, and to love itself.*

   Then visualize each *YHVH* יהוה joining each *ADNY* אדני of each cell so that every cell is *YAHDVNHY* יאהדונהי, male and female divine energies in balance. I often visualize the *ADNY* אדני letters as green. Purple and green are the healing colors of the healing angel Rafael.

7. Say, *I ask you, soul of each liver cell, to love the cell in which you reside. I love each soul of each liver cell. You are wonderful. Please inspire each cell to repair itself.*

8. Again see *YAHDVNHY* יאהדונהי in each cell. I often see it as alternating purple and green characters.

9. Then say, "I love each liver cell. I see each liver cell strong, well, and healthy. Strong cells . . . strong cells . . . (say eight times) . . . I see each liver cell very healthy. Healthy liver cells, healthy liver cells . . . healthy and wonderful liver (say ten times). Thank you, soul of my liver, for bringing healing. Thank you, soul of each liver cell, for bringing healthy repair and healing. Thank you God for giving me a healthy liver. I love you my liver. I love you my God."

Every morning, I go into my *mi'at meekdash,* my special room filled with volumes of books on Kabbalah and art. There, in the tradition of Chaim Vital and Rabbi Nachman of Breslov, I do *hitbodidut* prior to praying the traditional Jewish morning service. *Hitbodidut,* literally "seclusion," or "enclothement," is the traditional Hebrew word for "meditation." Rabbi Chaim Vital practiced it to achieve *Ru'ach HaKodesh* or the Holy Spirit. He went into seclusion, separating his soul from his body, disassociating from all corporeality, including corporeal thoughts.

Two hundred or so years later, Rabbi Nachman of Breslov created his own *hitbodidut* meditative experience based on Rabbi Chaim Vital's Kabbalistic practice. Rabbi Nachman would go into a secluded room and empty himself to God. He would talk with God about anything and everything.

This is the practice I do every morning. My doctor encouraged me to do this. He didn't know he was encouraging me to do *hitbodidut*, but he told me that, for my own health, I needed to "cry," to express my emotions. And who is better to express your emotions to than God?

In my special room, I visualize in front of me, in huge letters, *YHVH* יהוה. Or I visualize the Burning Bush, or a room filled with light. And I speak with these images with the same passion and trust that I would speak with my best friend. I first say aloud, *Ribbono shel Olam, Master of the Universe,* numerous times. This alters my level of consciousness. I then say *Ribbono shel Olam – Hineini, Master of the Universe, I am here to do whatever You want,* many times. After each time I say it, I visualize an experience that God and I succeeded in together — like when I met my wife immediately after praying for a wife; or the occasion of my being ordained as a rabbi; or the day we founded our synagogue; or the day we founded our seminary; or the many images of my sharing money with the homeless, doing God's work; or leading religious services. I then thank God for everything I have that I consider great or wonderful, and I mean *everything*.

I then begin to wrestle with God, argue with Him, fight with Him, even cry to Him when I can't understand why "bad things happen to good people." I then petition Him, often using meditations based on the Hebrew letters, knowing that certain letter sequences can be powerful software in helping to access the hardware of the Mind of God. For me this time of *hitbodidut* every morning, this "alone" time with God, is extremely valuable. It not only heightens and reinforces my relationship with God, it also greatly improves my technical ability as a prayer-person.

I have become so friendly toward and aware of God that I can almost *see* Him. And I believe that I now hear Him within. So, when I pray for people, He really is as close to me as the air I breathe. And I have every confidence that my healing prayer is working. If you want to be in the Greater Mind, the best advice I can give you is to talk to God every day. Set aside the same time every day to hear Him.

Many people ask if prayer has the same power over long distances as it does when you are in the same room with the person you are praying for.

I suspect that, theologically, every rabbi or priest would concede that it does — since prayer and God transcend space and time. I at least do believe healing prayer can be done at a distance, especially if you are praying for people you love who live in far-away towns or cities.

One of the remarkable properties of the *Sefirot,* or energy transformers, is their color. Each *Sefirotic* color has its own vibrational pattern and its own special energy. You can visualize different colors, corresponding to different *Sefirot,* surrounding people you know in different cities. Green and purple, for example, are very powerful in Kabbalistic healing. When we pray for someone far away, there is great efficacy in visualizing his or her injured leg being healed with these colors. They correspond with *Tiferet* (purple) and *Bina* (green), according to Cordovero's color system.

The *MiShibeirach* Prayer

There is a special healing prayer that Jewish people traditionally recite after the reading of the Torah. In some liberal synagogues, this prayer is said just before the reading of the Torah, or during other parts of the Sabbath service. This prayer is a holistic one calling for a *Refuah Shleimah,* a full (or complete) healing of body and soul. Either the rabbi or the prayer leader recites the names of the people who are ill in the synagogue community and asks that God bestow upon them a full healing. In our synagogue, our cantorial soloist, Charlene Brooks, and our signing choir, led by choir leader Nona Balk and Assistant Rabbi Shari Chen, lead us in this beautiful prayer of healing, the *MiShibeirach.*

MiShibeirach Avoteinu M'kor Hab'rachah l'imoteinu.
May He who blessed our Fathers be a source of blessing for our Mothers. May the Source of Strength who blessed all before us help us find the courage to make our lives a blessing, and let us say, amen.

To make the *MiShibeirach* even more efficacious, when we hear the names of those who are ill we should visualize each one of them healthy and well, standing before us. I often see the person in the beautiful green-purple light of healing. When your rabbi or minister or priest mentions the names of people who are ill, use the principle of the Greater Mind to bring healing. And remember a major tenet of Jewish healing — you are praying for not only the person called out by name, you are praying at this same time to give God strength. In distance prayer, we focus on how the *Shechina* suffers together with all those who suffer.

This is a sacred opportunity not only to pray to God but also *for* God. When we pray this kind of distance healing, we remind ourselves that we are all connected and that God lives within each one of us. It is She who is the connecting principle. Distance prayer in this way has power not only to bring healing to the person you are praying for — it also brings healing to the *Shechina*, the aspect of God that unites us all as one.

When I do either the Moses, Jeremiah, Aaron, or Hezekiah healing prayers for a person who is at a distance, I visualize that person standing right in front of me. When I pour healing light on her or him, with my hands or hand, it is as if I am pouring light on that person standing right there in the room.

The more distance healing you do, the more proficient you will be at it. The more healing prayer you do, the more powerful your imagination will be and the easier it will be for you to access the Greater Mind. Your prayers — short distance or long distance — will be more efficacious if you really believe that this is what God intends for you to do. That's why I emphasize that you do *hitbodidut* at least once every day, developing a strong friendship with God. You need to be in constant touch with the Creator, so that *Hashem* will work through you for healing again and again.

I do believe, however, that praying in the same room with the person you are praying for has *more* power. I understand this statement can be considered controversial, as it appears to diminish the power of God who transcends time and space. I don't mean to imply this. But when you and the person you are praying for are in the same room, you see her pain, you feel her love for you even more strongly and vividly — because you can see and hear her. As human beings, I think we are more influenced by seeing and hearing and touching. It's how God made us.

When I pray with people in front of the Holy Ark, some of them ask, "Is God more present here than He is by the roadside?" Yes and no, I say. God is just as present on the expressway or in the shopping center as He is by the Ark or altar. But, and this is a BIG but, we *feel* God's Presence more strongly near the sacred Torah scrolls. When we feel God's Presence more strongly, we pray with more *kavvanah*, we embrace the Greater Mind. And when we embrace the Greater Mind, prayer becomes the strongest power in the universe. I believe in distance prayer. I encourage distance prayer. But when you pray physically near the person you are praying for, it is almost as if you can see the Presence of God.

God bless you. And let *Hashem* be with you.

NOTES

1. Only some of these works are available in English. The Breslov Institute is currently working on an English translation of the complete work.

2. Rabbi Chaim Vital introduced this kind of silent secluded meditation — through which a person cures diseases of the soul, such as jealousy, depression, sadness, anger, and the lack of forgiveness — in his sixteenth-century classic *Sha'arei Kedusha* (Gates of Holiness). He called this meditative exercise *hitbodidut*. Through *hitbodidut*, we make ourselves available to receive *Ru'ach HaKodesh*. In order to achieve *Ru'ach HaKodesh* and practice *hitbodidut*, Vital instructs the meditator to achieve a state of perfect solitude by meditating alone in a house, secluded from any distractions, to such an extent as to separate soul, *Nefesh*, from the body. This first stage is a preparatory one, in which the goal is to achieve a state of perfect solitude. In the qualifying stage, the meditator then works to rid him- or herself of anger, sadness, and depression. When these sicknesses of the soul are removed, one is able to reach *Ru'ach HaKodesh*.

17

Love Is What You Need

WHEN I first came to Chicago to serve as rabbi of the new congregation we were developing, I found an apartment in the western suburbs. Subsequently, Peggy and I had to move seven times (it was the decade of the condo craze in Chicago) before we finally found a home we could call our own.

We found a beautiful leafy neighborhood where there were no less than two rabbis, three ministers, and one graduate theology student. One Thanksgiving, we all were invited to a neighbor's home, where the conversation inevitably turned to theology. One minister said to me, "Christianity is definitely Judaism's younger brother. But I also believe that there is more love in the New Testament than in the Old Testament."

I often have heard this said — to my great dismay. It is true that the word *love* appears more times in the New Testament than in the Old Testament. But the Hebrew scriptures balance this out by emphasizing love with great intensity.

I reminded my colleague that when something is rare, it is very precious. And when the Torah was written, love was an extremely holy word. Hence, the word love appears only in four commandments — two in the Book of Leviticus and two in the Book of Deuteronomy.

I explained to him that *hava*, Hebrew for love, does not refer here to the love a mother has for her son or daughter, or the romantic love between two people. When the Torah says:

You shall love your neighbor as yourself . . .

You shall love the stranger as yourself . . .

You shall love the Lord your God . . .

You shall love the stranger, for you were strangers in the land of Egypt . . .

it is speaking of a remarkable kind of love that can heal or inspire or bring together different peoples. The Torah takes "love" so seriously that, when it commands us to love the stranger, it is teaching us that the stranger is not really another person; the stranger is all of us, we ourselves.

Another of my minister friends was not satisfied with this explanation. He didn't believe that "love" in the Torah has the same force as it does in the New Testament. He gave as an example the Hebrew text *Ve'ahavta l're'akha kamokha* and said that the King James version of the Bible translates this text as "Thou shalt love thy neighbor as thyself" whereas the Jewish Publication Society Bible says, "Love your fellow as yourself."

The ministers asked if I knew the Aramaic translation, which would be closest to the language that Jesus spoke. I didn't know it by memory, but since I lived only a few houses away, I excused myself and retrieved my Rabbi's Bible with the second-century Aramaic version of Onkelos, an Aramaic scholar of that period. He translated the Hebrew into Aramaic as *U'terachameh l'chavrakh k'vatakh,* which would be: *And you shall love your friend as yourself.*

So here we were — two rabbis, three ministers, and a host with a graduate degree in Biblical Hebrew — trying to figure out, over turkey and cranberry sauce, is God commanding us to love our neighbor, our fellow, or our friend?

Our host recalled a text in Christian scripture in which Jesus declared to his students, "You have heard that it was said, *Ve'ahavta l're'akha kamokha* . . . You shall love your neighbor and hate your enemy. But I say to you, Love your enemies; and pray for those who persecute you. . . . For if you love those who love you, what reward do you have? Do not even the tax collectors do the same?" (Matthew 5:43–46).[1]

My host, in supporting the ministers, was saying that Jesus meant, "The rabbis think that the Torah's *Ve'ahavta l're'akha kamokha* means that you should love your *friends* as you love yourselves. But so what? Even the tax collector loves his friends." Therefore, my host said, "*Re'akha* doesn't mean just your friend. It also means *your fellow man.* So the Bible means we should love *everyone,* our enemies as well."

Were my friends correct in saying that love in the New Testament is more embracing than love in the Old Testament? Who was right?

When I got home that evening, I went to my Hebrew and English lexicon of the Old Testament, the classic by Brown, Driver, and Briggs. It defines the Hebrew word *re'akha* as "friend, companion, and fellow." So we all had a case. Both traditions recognize the importance of "love." Isn't that what really matters?

I also recalled a wonderful Hebrew Midrash that amends the Biblical text. It says *Ve'ahavta l're'akha kamokha,* which translates as "You shall love your fellow man because he is like you." This Midrash counsels us to "love your fellow man because, like you, God is within him." We are all made up of the stuff called God. If we acknowledge God within ourselves, and acknowledge God in the other, we will recognize that indeed we are all holographic. We all have the same spiritual DNA.

I have a very good friend who is a Baptist minister. To some extent, I am responsible for him entering the ministry. Before he did, he was my neighbor and worked at a small garage that serviced cars. One hot summer evening, we were sitting on my porch eating cherries and he asked, "How do you know if you're called to the ministry? Can God call you if you've done some bad things in your life? How do you know if you're worthy?"

I asked, "Do you feel an intense and wonderful closeness to God?"

He said, "Yes."

"Do you want God's forgiveness for your past? Do you intend to do good things from this day forward? Do you feel God has a purpose for you?" I asked him.

"Yes. He wants me to preach the gospel."

"Then accept that you are worthy. God is in all of us. If you feel called by God within every fiber of your being, then go for it."

And that's how Rick began his journey to become a preacher.

In some black traditions, the student minister or preacher studies texts and practices under his pastor. That's what Rick did. For a number of years, he studied and absorbed the Bible like a sponge. He was a natural.

I remember hearing him preach as a student minister. He was dynamic, as was the entire black Baptist service. The shouts from the congregation and the joy that was felt surely would have inspired the Baal Shem Tov.

The Torah says, "You are commanded to rejoice" (Deut. 16:15). Here was a church filled with Baptists clapping, singing, rejoicing, even following Torah. To paraphrase the word of Jacob, "The Lord was surely in this place." God surely is everywhere.

As Rick continued studying for the ministry, every so often he would visit me in my study at the synagogue and ask some Biblical questions. He and his wife Mary loved our healing services at the synagogue, and they would sometimes participate in our Wednesday night healing group. Now and then they would bring friends or offer up names in prayer.

In 1992, I founded the Hebrew Seminary of the Deaf (now called Hebrew Seminary). Since then, I have had the great privilege of ordaining other rabbis. This school is in part dedicated to training women and men to become rabbis who are fluent in sign language and can minister to both deaf and hearing Jews. It is also dedicated to the serious study and practice of Kabbalistic healing. I have ordained ten rabbis, including one who is profoundly deaf. Our ordination ceremony is very inspiring, but nothing could have prepared me for my friend Rick's ordination ceremony.

Whereas rabbis get ordained in their seminary, there is a Baptist tradition that a minister is ordained directly in the church — specifically in the church that he is about to serve. This was the case with my friend Rick.

Peggy and I received an invitation to witness the ordination and laying on of hands of the Reverend Rick. When the invitation came in the mail, it never occurred to me or Peggy that the hands laid on Rick's head during his ordination would be my very own.

In Reverend Rick's church, the tradition is that several different ministers from different churches are needed to lay on hands for the ordination. In addition, the ministerial candidate has to answer a host of theological questions. One is "If a single woman in your congregation calls you at 3 a.m. for emergency help, do you leave your bed of sleep and immediately go to her home? Do you go?" Rick immediately answered correctly, "Of course you go, but be sure to take your wife with you!"

Most of the other questions were more academic, relating to Christian scripture. I was quite surprised when the Church elders called my name and asked me to be the scorekeeper, to grade the answers. I protested, maintaining that the Hebrew Bible, not the Christian Bible, was my field of expertise. I was overruled. Then, I was given a sheet with all the questions and answers. I was now an expert. But not as much of an expert as Rick. He passed the test with close to a hundred percent of the right answers. But if I found this daunting, I clearly was not prepared for what happened next.

In the tradition of their church, ministers representing different churches in the area not only would ask Rick theological questions, they also would ordain him. They needed several ministers to lay on hands, but one of the preachers was not present and his absence was conspicuous. Again I heard my name called. "Rabbi Goldhamer, we would like you to be one of the ministers to ordain Rick Mercer into the ministry."

I accepted the call and put my hands on top of his head. Several other ministers put their hands on top of my hands. This was an enormous honor. Remember I was the only Jewish minister, a rabbi, in the whole church. Secondly, Rick is a dear, dear friend. What a joy it was for me to participate in his ordination.

Here we were — Rick, all the other ministers, and I — all touching to the extent that we became one vessel receiving the love of God. Even though this was a Christian ceremony ordaining a Christian minister in a black church, at the moment of ordination, I was not Jewish and they were not Christian. I was not white and they were not black. There was no *I* and there was no *they*. There was only *we*, and we were all One.

Christian scripture teaches in the Book of Mark that a fellow teacher approached Jesus and asked him to name the most important of all the Biblical commandments. Jesus answered, "The first of all the commandments is 'Hear O Israel, the Lord our God, the Lord is One'"[2] (Mark 12:28–33). Jesus meant by this that not only is there one God, but we are all one in Him. This is shown by a later statement of Jesus that the second most important commandment is, "Thou shalt love thy fellow as thyself," with the Midrashic meaning that your fellow is yourself.

Rabbi Abraham Heschel, the greatest twentieth-century Jewish theologian, wrote: "We never say three times a day in the *Sh'ma*, "Hear O Israel, the Lord our God, the Lord is perfect." Instead we say, "Hear O Israel, the Lord our God, the Lord is One." And one God means *no one* is ever alone. Rabbi Heschel was right. When my *zaidie* and I hugged, we became one. And when all of us put our hands together during Reverend Mercer's ordination, all of us became one with God. None of us was alone.

Clearly, it was unique for a rabbi to participate in the blessing and ordination of a black Baptist preacher. In that moment, we all felt so connected to one another that we all felt that we *were* one another. When we were of one heart, we all felt the power of God's love soaring through our veins. And we felt this because, at that moment, we were all intuiting a great truth: Each one of us is made up of every one of us. And love is the power that lets us see this.

We learn from a Hebrew commentary that a person cannot become a vessel for the Presence of God without first loving his or her fellow human beings. The Spirit of God cannot prosper amid discord and fighting; but when people love one another, that is when they receive God's blessings and Spirit. Only when we are of one heart can we attain that degree of spirituality that will allow us to receive God's light. We receive God's love most fully only when we recognize that we are all one.

Rick's ordination was late on a Sunday morning. That evening I was scheduled to speak to a synagogue men's group about God, healing, and my book *This Is for Everyone.* The rabbi of the synagogue made it clear to me that there were three other people on the panel and that I only had seven minutes to speak. I had a text prepared on the power of faith; but after being part of Rick's ordination and seeing all the ministers of different religions and different colors coming together with one heart, I realized that the most important topic for me to discuss was *Love.* I wanted to tell them that God's blessings flow into us most powerfully when people come together with one heart in love.

We might be fluent in different spiritual practices or be mavens in meditative practice. We might have enormous faith in God and in God's healing powers. Our ability to visualize and imagine might be operating on a high level. But if we don't have *Love*, the chance of our being a spiritual channel for God's healing is nil. This is why the Hebrew word *gilgul* (incarnation of a soul in a body) has the same *gematria* as the Hebrew word *Chesed* (loving kindness). Kabbalah is teaching in this that God's healing spiritual energy can flow through us to the person we are praying for, if we love him/her and if we recognize that we are essentially of one heart. That is, we are one. The power of love is a great Kabbalistic healing secret.

This teaching about love as a secret to healing can be found in the second book of the Hebrew Bible, the Book of Exodus, Chapter 15, which I discussed in this book's Preface. I believe this passage is the cornerstone for Jewish medical practice. And by "Jewish medical practice," I mean Kabbalistic healing. "He said, if you will heed the Lord your God diligently, doing what is upright in His sight, giving ear to His commandments and keeping all His laws, then I will not bring upon you any of the diseases . . ."

The word translated as commandments here is *mitzvot. Mitzvot* includes not only ritual and legal deeds, but also ethical commandment, to the extent that, in the Jewish community, people loosely translate *mitzvot* as "good deeds." This scripture shows clearly that there is an ethical correlation between health and illness. Health is connected to right action. Illness happens when we deny right action in our lives.

There can be no real healing without bringing in the moral context of a person's illness. It's not enough for physicians to treat patients only by treating a diseased bladder or a ruptured appendix. The patient must be treated holistically. The patient's soul must be probed and prodded with the same vigor as his or her physical body.

HOW TO: Hugging Love Meditation Leading to Healing

Here is a wonderful "Love" meditation that I do often. It is very simple, based on Oneness. In this meditation, I and the person I pray with stand in front of the open Ark, recognizing that we are standing on holy ground. (Holy ground does not have to be in front of an Ark — it can be anywhere you feel God's Presence.) In this sacred awareness, we hug. And we hug some more. And then we hug even more.

As incredible as this seems, I have seen that hugging with love in this way leads to healing. Of course, the person who is ill needs to accept medical treatment and take the prescribed medicines. But in combination with that, hugging regularly on holy ground — with faith and love and with the internal dynamic that the person who needs help is receiving healing from God — truly leads to healing.

As we hug, I recognize that we are not really separate but are both made of the same stuf, and that stuff is God. When our souls come together as we hug, we both feel *Chesed* — the love that we have for the person we are hugging and for ourselves. Feeling the tremendous love, we both recite two texts again and again.

The first is: *Hear O Israel, the Lord our God, the Lord is One.* This verse teaches us that not only is God One, not only is God One in us, but we are one in God. We are never alone; we are always one with the other.

The second text we recite again and again as a mantra is: *You shall love your fellow as you love yourself.* As we recite we remember that this means: You shall love your fellow because he/she is like yourself, made up of the stuff of God.

In Chapter 1, we learned that *gematria* teaches that *Ahava,* the Hebrew word for love, has the numerical equivalent of 13. And *YHVH*, the most powerful Presence of God has the numerical equivalent of 26. Therefore, when *two* people hug and love (13 + 13 = 26), the Presence of God and God's light automatically join them.

It's not that God says, "Ah, now that they are hugging in love, I will reward them with My Presence." God's Presence automatically, necessarily, emerges into our awareness when two people hug in love. God can't help but exist when two people embrace this way: 13 + 13 is always 26. *Ahava* plus *Ahava* is always *YHVH*.

And this is exactly what happened when we ministers blessed Rick with one heart. The Presence of God was powerfully present in love.

HOW TO: Love Your Neighbor Meditation Delivering Divine Healing Energy

1. Sit opposite your friend. You in one seat and your friend in another, facing each other.

2. Visualize with your eyes closed a beam of gold/white healing light/ energy coming down from the heavens, through the room, onto the crown of your head, *Keter.*

3. Inhale gently but deeply through your nostrils so that, as you breathe in, the light is activated and travels through *Keter* into your heart, *Tiferet.*

4. Hold your breath for three to four seconds and visualize your heart filled with light.

5. As you breathe out through your nostrils, silently say, "You shall love the Lord your God with all your heart, with all your soul, and with all your might." Also visualize your heart opening up, especially when you say the word "heart," and the gold/white healing light/ energy of your heart flowing from your heart through the air into your friend, filling every single cell of his/her body with gold/white healing light/energy. See or feel every cell in your friend's body — every cell — receiving healing light/energy. View yourself as a vessel of divine healing energy.

6. Again, visualize the beam of gold/white healing light light/energy coming down from the heavens, through the roof, onto *Keter,* your crown and moving down through *Keter* into *Tiferet,* your heart area.

7. Hold your breath for three to four seconds, and see your heart filled with divine light/energy.

8. As you exhale through your nostrils, say silently to yourself as before, "You shall love the Lord your God with all your heart, with all your soul and with all your might" . . . but this time when you say "heart" and visualize your heart opening up, visualize the divine light/energy flowing through the air into every cell of your friend's *affected organ or area.* Visualize the whole organ filled with shining light. Know that every cell of the organ is being transformed to a healthy cell. Feel confident that healing is taking place. See the affected organ filled with the divine light energy and know that you are a vessel of higher healing energy from God.

9–11. Repeat steps 6–8.

12. As you are seeing the affected organ or area filled with healing light/ energy, see on it also *YHVH* יהוה, the name of God, in different colors: First see the letters in white, then in purple, and finally in green. Each of these holy letters is a powerful form of divine energy.

13. After seeing *YHVH* יהוה on the affected area in the three colors, hold your friend's hands with love, be aware of how much you love her or him, and refresh your awareness that God lives in your friend. Ask God to heal your friend's affected organ. Tell God how much you love your friend, and how good your friend is, and why she/he should be healed.

14. Remember God lives in your friend. Understand why you are commanded "You shall love the Lord your God, with all your heart, with all your soul and with all your might." When you pray with this understanding, you are praying not only for your friend, you are also praying for *Adonai* — God who lives in your friend. God also needs our prayers. And where do we find God? Within each one of us.

15. Then visualize your friend completely well. Remember: Pray as if your prayer is already answered. See her/him doing an activity she couldn't do, when she/he was ill. *And thank God for having healed her/him.*

Every morning before I meditate, I do my daily prayers. I invoke the Presence of God, perhaps by visualizing a Burning Bush or the whole room filled with light and blazing with the Hebrew letters *YHVH* יהוה. I see them in glistening white characters. I know the face of God is behind the light. But it is impossible for me to see Her/Him. I only see clearly the *YHVH* יהוה, the face of God.

Every day I thank God that I am healthy and well. I thank God for the miracle of my life, my wonderful wife, the wonderful books all around me, my good name, and the honor of serving as a rabbi who practices Kabbalistic healing. I also thank God for what *Hashem* has helped me accomplish this past week, this past year, and through the course of this lifetime. I let God know how much I love Him with all my heart.

Rabbi Yaakov shared with me a profound secret about how a person can awaken or stir his or her love of God — begin by examining the kindnesses that God is constantly giving to you. I always ask the people with whom I pray to write a list of the gifts and kindnesses that they receive every day and every week from God. I advise them to then meditate on them, until they feel the incredible and personal love that God constantly shows them. After you have done this, imagine how it would feel if you were God, and you were the constant giver of these gifts. You will see even more clearly the great love that God has for you. This very deep secret comes from the Kabbalistic book *Tanya*.

Kabbalah teaches that we are to love God with all of our higher divine soul, *Nefesh Elohit, and* with our lower animalistic soul, *Nefesh Behamit.* "As above, so below; as below, so above." This also means that whatever we do down here, God reflects back to us. When the great healing rabbi, the Baal Shem Tov, was asked to comment on this, he said this means that God is your mirror. This Kabbalistic secret derives from the Hebrew Bible: "As face answers to face in water, so does one man's heart to another" (Proverbs 27:19). The same principle applies to the heart. One who loves God with all his heart will receive that love reflected back to him.

The intensity of our love for God that we express in words and actions will be reflected back to us by God. We should constantly open up our hearts to feel His Presence, through prayer and through action. As we make a concentrated effort to open up our hearts to God, we will be divinely blessed with God's opening His heart to us. In our "Love Your Neighbor Meditation," we literally open up our heart to God who lives in our fellow human being.

We learn several Kabbalistic secrets of healing in these mystical teachings. We learn that there is a correlation between acts of love and healing. We learn that health is connected to our carrying out ethical commandments and that illness is connected to abandoning an ethical way of life. We learn that God is not only the great Healer, but also our mirror: "As above, so below; as below, so above." We learn that the more we extend love to God, people, and animals, the more God's love will be reflected back on us, which will lead to great spiritual health. *Love of God and love of people is a huge component of Kabbalistic healing.*

NOTES

1. *The Jewish Annotated New Testament,* Amy-Jill Levine and Marc Zvi Brettler, eds. (Oxford University Press: New York, 2011).

2. In Judaism, this prayer is referred to as the *Sh'ma* prayer.

The Luz Bone:
God's Antidote to Depression

ONE of the miracles I've experienced during my many years in Chicago is the miracle of Gallaudet University. I'm still amazed, and more than inspired, that it was during Abraham Lincoln's tenure as president of the United States that this remarkable university was founded. This is a school where all classes, up to and including the Ph.D. level, are taught in American Sign Language. It is an amazing sight to go into the cafeteria at lunch time and see hands waving in all directions, communicating with precision and beauty the intricate details of chemical engineering, Greek philosophy, and American history via American Sign Language.

I had the good fortune of being offered a professorship at Gallaudet one year. It was one of the most wonderful times of my life. I taught courses in philosophy and met deaf students from all over the world. I even met someone who was considering creating a university like Gallaudet in Russia, and several professors who were interested in my work in healing.

It was because of my connection to Gallaudet that I met Rabbi Dr. Yaakov Dresher. I remember studying with him many times. One time Peggy came with me to Washington, and we both visited Rabbi Dresher and his family. We were sitting at the dining room table with some of Rabbi Yaakov's students when Rabbi Yaakov asked me, "*Nu* Douglas, how is it going with your praying?"

I shared with him that I loved praying both alone and with people, and that in recent years I had been studying Rabbi Nachman of Breslov's (1772–1810) works on prayer. Rabbi Yaakov asked, "Do you enjoy Rabbi Nachman's writings?"

I answered that I thoroughly enjoyed the healing lessons in *Likutei*

Moharan. I especially learned a lot from a unique theme in his text that every organ in the human body possesses an inherent spiritual power or soul, and the functions of that organ or limb correlate to that specific soul. Rabbi Yaakov was glad that I admired and was studying one of his heroes. He reminded me, though, that even though Rabbi Nachman was a great healer, he personally suffered bouts of depression. Fortunately, he also knew a Kabbalistic secret that brings happiness.

I told Rabbi Yaakov that I knew Rabbi Nachman maintained that *Hashem* is within each of us, and has a purpose for each of us, and that acknowledging this would help us greatly in fighting our personal demons. But what, I wondered, is his Kabbalistic secret for happiness?

Before I could say more, Rabbi Dresher began telling a story, written by Rabbi Nachman. Once upon a time, a long time ago, there was a poor Jewish man named Ezra who earned a living by digging clay. After many months of digging and digging, he unearthed what appeared to him to be a rare and valuable precious gem — perhaps a diamond. He took the stone to a jeweler, who told him to take it to London, where he would be able to get it properly appraised and sold.

Ezra couldn't afford the trip to London. He sold everything he had to raise funds for a ticket, but he still didn't have enough money. So he went to the captain of the nearest ship that was traveling to London and showed him his amazing find. The captain was a very salty gentleman who knew little of culture and the delicacies of life. But when he saw the large jewel, he was enormously impressed, offered Ezra a first-class room, and treated him like a wealthy gentleman.

Every morning, afternoon, and evening, Ezra took his meals at a little table facing the sea, with the precious jewel in front of him as he ate. This cheered him up enormously. He felt so happy. Actually, he had never felt as happy as he was since he found the stone. For two weeks, Ezra enjoyed his travels, imagining the large amount of money he would receive for his precious jewel, and how he would pay the captain what he owed him and still have much money left over. These were his daydreams morning, afternoon, and night.

One morning, as he was having breakfast with his precious jewel in front of him, Ezra fell asleep. The busboy came to his table while he was sleeping and thought he was finished eating. So he cleared the table, throwing the crumbs as well as the precious stone all into the sea.

When Ezra woke up and saw what had happened, his joy was instantly transformed to sadness and fright. How would he pay for the trip? The captain might kill him, if he doesn't pay what he owes. What's the purpose of the trip if he has no precious jewel to sell?

Suddenly, it was as if *Hashem* whispered words of wisdom to Ezra: Almost instantly, he realized that if he embraced a depressed disposition, confessing his tale of woes to the burly captain, he would be thrown over the edge of the boat. So Ezra decided to embrace the Greater Mind.

He had studied some *hasidut* literature and realized that if he embraced *Mohin de Gadlut* and became happy, this would not only fool the captain but would also activate *Hashem*'s Presence within him completely. So, instead of risking that the captain would throw him overboard, he threw his worries, his Lesser Mind, *Mohin de Katnut* overboard and embraced the Greater Mind. He was happy and showed happiness day and night, as if nothing had happened. When you are in the Greater Mind, nothing bad can happen to you.

One day the captain approached Ezra, whom he still thought was a very wealthy man, and asked if he, the captain, could buy a large quantity of wheat in Ezra's name, since he himself didn't have the money to pay for it. The captain knew that when he arrived in London, he would be able to sell the wheat at a great profit and make a lot of money. Ezra, trusting in the Greater Mind, and showing great joy and confidence, agreed to the deal. As the ship docked in the London harbor, the captain died, and Ezra inherited a great profit, worth many times more than the precious jewel!

Rabbi Nachman concludes his tale by explaining that the precious stone never belonged to Ezra. That's why it did not remain with him. The wheat was meant to be his, and that's why it did remain with him. Ezra got what he deserved because he remained happy, because he embraced the Greater Mind.

Rabbi Yaakov taught us that morning that it is up to us to be always in the Greater Mind, even when things look bad. Even when things look awful. We need to embrace the Greater Mind, and kick out the Lesser Mind. We need to embrace thinking happy, being happy, and acting happy.

It's not magic, but it's close to it. When we embrace the Greater Mind of happiness, we activate the Presence of God within us. With God, only good can follow.

Ezra forced himself to be happy. That's okay. It's not only okay, it's great. Force happiness and genuine joy will appear. "Fake it 'til you make it."

After Rabbi Dresher shared this wonderful story about being happy and embracing the Greater Mind, we were all touched and moved greatly, except my wife Peggy. She said, "Rabbi Dresher, I love your story, but sometimes when someone is depressed, even a moving story like this doesn't help. Some people don't have the wherewithal, the inner strength, to overcome depression. They don't feel they have anything within them that can give them hope. What do we do then?"

Rabbi Dresher said, "According to the *Zohar*, we learn that when the Messiah arrives and the Resurrection begins, the physical body will rise and be revitalized on the merit of a single bone in your body that does not decay in the grave. It remains intact. This bone is called the Luz bone. The Talmud teaches that *Hashem* will resurrect the entire body through this bone that is within each one of us." He further told Peggy that the eighteen blessings of the *Amidah* prayer correspond to the first eighteen vertebrae in the spine. And located next to the eighteenth vertebrae is a small spinal vertebrae called the Luz. The Luz bone corresponds to the nineteenth blessing of the *Amidah* prayer. Dr. Dresher also told me that different medieval sources disagreed as to the location of this resilient bone — some writers said it is in the tailbone or coccyx area; others indicate that it is at the base of the neck. The important fact, though, is that it exists.

After death and burial, he said, the entire human body decays except for this tiny vertebra, this one bone. It is indestructible. It does not decay in any way and cannot be consumed by fire. It exists in every human being. The Luz bone will serve as the building block from which *Hashem* will build the body anew, at the time of the Resurrection of the Dead.

Rabbi Dresher then said to all of us, "When a person has fallen into a deep state of depression, and he feels that he is 'dead,' there is one way we can encourage him to sit with us and do healing prayer. This is to remind them that no matter how deep the hole is that the person has fallen into, no matter how dead the person feels, we need to remind him or her that there exists an indestructible part in him that will form the basis for a new life, a new resurrection — the Luz bone.

This Luz bone is spoken of as the part of God within a person. When we recognize that we are not separate selves, that we are part of God and God is part of us, then we will begin to know our purpose and our meaning in life. We need to inspire the person who is depressed to recognize that she is part of God, through this amazing nineteenth vertebra, the Luz bone.

I realize that the spinal anatomy as related in the Talmud does not correspond with our modern medical model, which Rabbi Yaakov most certainly knew. But the notion of working with the Luz bone in this way has proven so useful in healing practice that the story retains power. What is essential is the recognition that there is something in us that is indestructible, part of the whole, and divine.

HOW TO: How to Inspire Someone Who Is Depressed to Embrace the Greater Mind — and to Discover that Healing Prayer Is Worthwhile

The purpose of this meditation is not to unchain the person from the chains of depression, but to ask that person to make him- or herself ready for prayer. Here is my instruction to the depressed person:

1. Focus on your breath. Just be aware of breathing in and out.

2. Focus on your Luz bone. You can even touch it. In my healing practice, I have found it very useful to consider that it is the coccyx.

3. Recognize that this is your Essence. This is your indestructible part. There is no sin, no misfortune, no tragedy that can erase who you are. Recognize that God loves you so much that just as your Luz bone, so your essence will always be there. God will always allow you to find a way out of this awful depression, because the Luz bone is that concrete bit of God within you. The Luz bone shows that you are not a separate self cut off from God.

4. Again, focus on your Luz bone. Bind yourself to it. Concentrate on it. Know that this bone, this amazing bit of bone and bit of God is the door to your happiness. Touch your Luz bone again and focus on it again. This is God's way of saying "You are indestructible and I will transform and resurrect you, from great great sadness to great great joy, through healing prayer."

Rabbi Nachman of Breslov always taught that the most important cure for any illness, especially mental depression, is turning to God — what the spiritual community calls *teshuvah* or "turning." Each one of us has a bit of God within us. When we recognize with *Mohin de Gadlut*, the Greater Mind, that God is within us from head to toe, then we have no fear of events that may befall us.

Rabbi Levi Yitzhak maintains that if you are in a sad state or if you are depressed, you need to embrace the Greater Mind. Then you will have no fear or anxiety. You will have no depression.

A person who is greatly depressed is denying that God is the fundamental Reality, of which he/she is a part. The *Sefirot* in that person are in a state of imbalance. This puts him/her in the *Mohin de Katnut,* the Lesser Mind. One who is in the Lesser Mind in this way is preoccupied with the limited life of the ego, to the extent of ignoring that he/she is part of the Greater Life of the Whole. When disconnected in this way from the light of God, the person is in what the ancients spoke of as a state of sin.

When I use the word "sinner" in this context, I don't mean a morally repugnant individual who cheats and steals, though such a person is surely a sinner. By sin here, I mean an activity which separates us from God and creates a vacuum, an emptiness, even a state of darkness, which forces us to be totally preoccupied with the limited life of the Ego. And into this vacuum of disconnection, depression creeps.

When someone is disconnected from God, he/she allows negative energy to enter generally, and perhaps even into a specific area of the body. We use the positive energy of the Hebrew letters in sequences to counter this negative energy. Sometimes the *Shiviti* prayer using the monthly permutations of *YHVH* is quite effective because, if negative energy has entered into a specific area of the body, this healing meditation will bring the different energy centers of the ill person into spiritual balance. She/he then becomes quite receptive to the next step in the healing process.

Alternatively, we might use permutations of the *Tetragrammaton,* the Ineffable Name, or bringing together male and female energies through a union of the Holy One and His *Shechina*. The Hebrew letters are codes, sacred codes of energy that allow us to treat disease caused by misalignment of spiritual energies. Misalignment can cause corruption in the spiritual DNA of brain cells in the temporal lobes, and the result is depression.

I remember praying with a young woman many years ago when I first recognized the power of prayer in healing. She was the nineteen-year-old daughter of a couple in my synagogue who told me she was suffering from depression. She was seeing a psychiatrist and a psychologist, but her depression persisted. I prayed with her once a week for almost two months, but she still continued to be depressed.

I shared my dilemma with Rabbi Daniel Dresher. He began by teaching me the meaning of the word depression. He asked me how often I filled the tires in my car with air. I told him I never fill my tires; my wife Peggy is in charge of auto maintenance. He seemed a little perturbed when I said that, but said, "You do know that when a tire on your car — or any tire — loses its air, that tire is called a 'depressed' tire? This means that the air has escaped the tire and now it is deflated."

He then said, "According to the Kabbalah, when you have a leaking of the divine from within you, to the extent that you are deflated of God, you become depressed."

The young woman I was praying with had an eating disorder. No matter how hard she tried, it appeared to her that she was gaining rather than losing weight. On top of that, her closest girlfriend had died in a car accident the year before. Here was a young female college student whose body-image was very poor and whose closest confidant had been snatched away. It was as if the divine had leaked out of her. She was spiritually deflated. She did not feel at all the Presence of God within her.

Rabbi Dresher urged me to use specific spiritual healing modalities to fill this young woman up once again with the feeling that God was in her still from head to toe. She needed to be in the Greater Mind. That is when her depression will leave, he said. Now, twenty years later, this young woman practices medicine in Chicago. She is married and has two children, and continues to be filled with the Presence of God.

I often see people who are depressed or suffering from terrible anxiety. Even though they see a therapist regularly and receive medicines from their psychiatrist — which definitely helps — they are still depressed. That's why I believe that it is crucial that the person who is suffering from depression abandon his or her preoccupation with the limited life of the ego and embrace the greater life of the Whole of God. When he diverts his preoccupation from a limited life of failures and successes and more failures, to a complete life teaching that everything is God, everything is in God, and God is in everything, including himself, he is on the road to recovery. This is a great secret of Kabbalistic healing.

Depression is not just unhappiness. It is extreme unhappiness to the extent that it is a kind of helplessness. Everything around us and within us is of no value. The Kabbalah teaches that the Creator created each life to be happy. Each one of us, each one of our lives is meant to be happy and have a purpose. We are not only made up of blood, bones, sinews, flesh, muscles, and organs, but every one of us is made up of the stuff of God. Each of us is made up of the Light of God.

Then why are so many people depressed? If each of us is made up of the Light of God, whose very nature is to share and to give and to be happy, why are so many people depressed?

Because we don't turn on the Light of God that is within us. We fail to flip the switch so that the light can shine in us. We don't inflate the depressed tire within us.

We have learned well from Rabbi Nachman of Breslov that there are correlations between body and soul and that everything is holographic. Everything contains within it the ten *Sefirot*. Every organ or limb is made up of ten *Sefirot*, and so is soul. We know now that with his method, when we do healing of any organ, or any limb, or any part of the body, we need to speak directly to its soul. This is his key teaching and a powerful secret of Kabbalistic healing. We call this kind of meditation "Soul Healing" or "Soul Re-pair."

We human beings share all life, including our own life, with the Divine. Each one of us shares the life we live on Earth with God. We are a pair, each one of us is part of a pair comprised of the divine and the human fused together. When we know this Secret, we are in the Greater Mind. When we don't know this secret, we are susceptible to despair. When we lack the enlightenment that we and God are a pair, we embrace despair and need re-pair.

Re-pair what? We need to re-pair our *Mohin de Katnut*, our Lesser

Mind, and change it to *Mohin de Gadlut,* the Greater Mind. We need to become aware of our divinity; we need to realize that the potential within us is unlimited. We need to repair our *Mohin de Katnut,* so that we can see how unique and special we are.

The psychiatrist and therapist begin this process with mood elevators and talk therapy. This is wonderful. But we teachers of the Kabbalah continue their therapies by re-pairing the relationship of the sick person with God. We do this through different modalities of healing prayer.

Kabbalah teaches that each one of us has come into this world with a purpose, to perfect our souls. We do this governed by karma and *hashgaha pratit,* God's supervising and super-loving providence for each one of us. We come here to correct the deficiencies of our souls. When we have done this, when we ultimately perfect our souls, our complete connection to the Light of God will have been achieved.

Happiness is ours to embrace. But if we have created sin through wrong choices and bad actions in this life, in past lives, we have created a space between ourselves and the Light of God. And into this void creeps the dangerous depression. When that happens, we need to see that our disconnection from God is a fundamental cause of our depression and anxiety.

If we were in the Greater Mind, we would feel God's love for us and God's purpose for us. We would see love and purpose in the world around us. But if our soul does not feel this love, this purpose, this God, and instead feels despair and depression, there is a correction or *tikkun* that needs to be made at the level of our soul. This *tikkun* is made through prayer and through sacred cellular energy techniques.

We learned in Chapter 12 that illness is rooted in the distortion of energetic information in our cells. Any disease, like depression, must be characterized by the breakdown of rhythmic behavior in the cells. Everything in the universe, including us, has to function in a rhythmic fashion to sustain itself. Breakdowns in this rhythmic behavior cause illness. We repair this breakdown by doing a form of Soul Repair — because illness originates not only at the cellular level, but *with the soul of each cell.*

Cells are always vibrating, contracting and expanding, transforming matter to energy and energy to matter. When cells contract, it is as if they are breathing out; when they expand, it's as if they are breathing in. According to Kabbalah, if cells contract too much or don't expand enough, or if they expand too much, we have a distortion in the rhythmic behavior of the cells, which leads to various illnesses, for example cancer or chronic fatigue syndrome.

Kabbalah and Kabbalistic healing focus on Balance. We strive for the middle column, for *Tiferet*, for Balance. Imbalance results from a breakdown of the rhythmic behavior of cells. When a cell was first conceived, before it differentiated into a kidney cell or a liver cell, etc., that cell was in an undifferentiated state or stem cell state. It was in a state whose code or sequence of Hebrew energies was pure and well. To repair or heal a cell in either rhythmic behavior dysfunction or distortion of information dysfunction, we visualize that cell in its original sequence of letters/energies. This is similar to "restoring" your computer to a previous date, when you want to correct a problem with it. We bring this healing down from above. This is what the Kabbalah means when it teaches "God created healing before God created the world."

How do we bring a cell back to its original state, its stem-cell-like state? We transform its soul back to the undifferentiated state that preceded negative energy and disease by applying Hebrew-letter codes appropriate to its cellular structure. When we apply the codes of the Hebrew letters to different cellular structures, we can achieve Kabbalistic healing. This is another profound Kabbalistic secret of healing

We know that depression can result from too much or too little activity in the brain's temporal lobes, in addition to too much activity in the deep limbic system. In depression, nerve cells don't present enough neurotransmitters. When balance is disturbed, behavior, mood, and thought are compromised and we have depression. With regard to depression, each cell in the temporal lobes needs to be in a state of balance. This means that the Hebrew letters/energies that inform each cell need to be in balance not only within its own cell but also with every other cell. This is a major secret of Kabbalistic healing.

In my practice as a rabbi helping with depression, I have seen that it is of utmost importance to return the temporal lobe cells to the pure state they were in before negative energies overwhelmed them. The cellular structure in the individual cell of the temporal lobes is made up of the energies of *Adonai*, which puts each temporal lobe cell in a vulnerable situation. By embracing only the *Shechina* energies and not also the transcendent *Hashem* energies, the cell is now in a state of imbalance. By helping the cell embrace male and female divine energies in a balanced way, we can pour God's healing light onto every temporal lobe cell so that it can become once again healthy and vibrant.

The following text was written by Professor Ann Morris, a good friend and colleague whose daughter suffered from severe depression. Her daughter did very well when we combined medical and spiritual Kabbalistic therapies to remove her pain and suffering. Dr. Morris was overjoyed at the results and I asked her if she would write a brief description of her daughter's experience.

Two years ago, my own family became one of those in need. Our world was pulled from its healthy roots and lost equilibrium. My thirty-something daughter fell into the despair associated with the mental health diagnosis of "major depressive disorder." Since college, she experienced episodes of severe sadness and anxiety treated by talk therapy and short-term psychotropic medications. Her psychiatrist predicted that as she aged, the disorder's severity could exponentially expand. His medical precision predicted the devastating nightmare that eventually became reality.

My daughter became isolated and could not work or be left alone due to sudden panic attacks. In-patient psychiatric hospitalization after the first suicide attempt left her catatonic due to the multiple number of medications tried and failed. The second suicide attempt occurred just days after she begged me "to just let her go." Believing that dying was the only option to relieve the pain, she overdosed on her prescribed medications, but luckily medical experts saved her life.

My life at that time was narrow and regimented — acting and feeling only according to my daughter's medical condition. I did not even call Rabbi Goldhamer for support. He however, characteristically reached out to me and suggested with insistence and energy that we encourage my daughter to incorporate healing prayer as another treatment protocol. He carefully explained how Kabbalistic healing techniques complement Western medical practices, focusing directly on the forebrain's frontal lobe, temporal lobe, and the limbic system to ease depression symptoms.

Open and hopeful, my daughter welcomed Rabbi and his wife Peggy's hospital visits to support and explain the healing process. A trusting connection existed between them from her childhood that sparked a faintness of hope to begin the parallel process of ECT (electroconvulsive therapy), medication, talk therapy, and healing prayers. I believe with certainty that a strong engagement with the healer is an essential element in the method's success.

Our learning curve in conducting these healing prayers was initially quite high, but after three months, the process became a comfort and friend. Incremental improvements appeared as she completed clinical treatments, individual healing sessions with Rabbi Goldhamer and our Assistant Rabbi Shari Chen. After one year, she was able to resume her life, slowly recapturing her career and beginning an advanced degree.

It has been two and a half years since Rabbi Goldhamer joined our team, his specialty enormously contributing to a more positive outcome. As a result, my daughter is experiencing a more balanced, productive, and happy life. I believe, with great conviction, that Rabbi Goldhamer's gifts in healing wisdom and goodness have all been monumental in reaching this outcome. Working respectively, we found that no one treatment truly fits all. Thank you, Rabbi, for teaching us that God is in each of us, encouraging every person to care for others and to contribute to positive change.

I have learned that divine light or energy that we receive into our hands can be delivered to patients suffering depression as an excellent supplement to talk therapy and chemistry. As I pour divine light onto the temporal lobe cells, I practice Rabbi Nachman's healing modality. I speak silently to the souls of the cells of the patient, asking those souls to encourage the cells in which they reside to repair themselves, to heal themselves and love themselves. There is great benefit in learning to speak to the souls of the cells, tell them you love them . . . tell each temporal lobe cell that you love it. Repeat many times à la Rabbi Nachman, "Strong cells, strong cells happy cells, happy cells . . . joyous cells, joyous cells . . . happy cells, happy cells . . . healthy temporal lobe cells."

In keeping with the Law of Sympathetic Vibration, cells spoken to in this manner vibrate more strongly and are more energetic. Other cells in the temporal lobes will adopt these healthy vibrational patterns.

Since the first great *tzimtzum*, when God contracted and then expanded, such rhythm became the pattern of the universe, constantly contracting and expanding. Kabbalah recognizes that, to be healthy, there must be a balance between the breathing in and breathing out activity of every cell. Balance is the key to good health. This is a key Kabbalistic principle. The Arizal prayer book teaches that the Silent Prayer (*Amidah*) blessing for healing corresponds to the *Sefira* of *Tiferet*, Balance. All of the different Silent Prayer blessings correspond to different *Sefirot*.

HOW TO: Eliminate Mental Depression by Lifting the *Shechina* out of Her Exile

Here is a vision in which the healer focuses on the joyous, healthy happy nature of each cell and on three flowing beams of light. It is essential for the healer to recognize with focused *kavvanah* that the divine light from above that is being delivered to each cell has within it the *Sefirotic* energy of *Tiferet* — Balance — enabling the cells to be in a constant state of Balance when contracting and expanding. The healer must be vividly aware of three flows of divine energy — one from the heavens onto *Keter* (crown of the head), one from the heavens onto the left palm, and one from the heavens onto the right palm . . . and then how two flows leave his/her hands and enter into the temporal lobes of the sick person. Rabbi Dresher always taught me, "*Where attention goes, energy flows.*"

1. You (the healer) and your friend sit down, preferably both facing east, but this is not mandatory.

2. Be comfortable. Be aware of your breathing. Feel the rhythmic breathing behavior of breathing in, deeply and gently, and breathing out, deeply and gently.

3. As you breathe in and out, feel the Presence of God strongly. If

you are outside, look at the mountains, trees, sky. If you are inside, recognize that it is not an accident that you are doing this healing for your friend. Have you considered that this might be a purpose in your life? Feel your connection to God.

4. While your friend continues to sit, you stand up and lift your arms into the air at about shoulder height, with palms facing the heavens. Visualize three beams of light: One beam of gold/white light comes from the heavens onto *Keter,* the crown of your head, a second beam of gold/white light comes down onto the palm and fingers of the left hand, and a third beam of gold/white light comes down onto the palm and fingers of the right hand. The central beam of light, coming into the crown of your head, is filled with many purple sets of *YHVH* יהוה.

5. Now stand behind the individual receiving healing, with your left palm and fingers facing the person's left temporal lobe and the right palm and fingers facing his/her right temporal lobe. Visualize light coming out of the left hand into the left temporal lobe and light coming out of the right hand into the right temporal lobe.

6. Breathe in through your nostrils, gently and deeply. As you do this, activate the middle column so that the middle column of light filled with purple sets of *YHVH* יהוה moves into *Tiferet,* your heart, and fills it with many purple sets of *YHVH* יהוה.

7. As you breathe out deeply and gently, visualize light with many sets of *YHVH* יהוה. flowing from your heart through both arms and out your fingers and palms, into the cells of the temporal lobes of the person you are praying for.

8. Each temporal lobe cell already has feminine energies *ADNY* אדני or *Shechina.* Visualize the masculine *YHVH* sets coming out of your hands and joining with the feminine *ADNY* in every cell, healing and transforming the feminine code to a balanced code of יאהדונהי, so that every cell of the temporal lobes returns to its original sacred code of balanced energy of good health. Making this your inner thought allows you to be a healing instrument of God, bringing every temporal lobe cell back to its original pristine state before it was damaged by imbalanced energies.

9. Thank God for giving you the sacred privilege to do this. Thank God for allowing your friend to be well. See your friend well and happy.

10. Repeat steps 4–9 two more times. On the final time, be more elaborate with your own language as you conclude your prayer, thanking God from the bottom of your heart for healing your friend.

HOW TO: Eliminate Mental Depression Using the Healing Modality of Rabbi Hezekiah

I recognize that not everyone has his own *shul* or *bima* or Holy Ark. But if you are praying for someone on a regular basis to alleviate depression, do this prayer (as any other healing prayer) in a sacred place that you consider to be special. Outdoors is perfectly fine, but the area must allow you the wherewithal to feel the Presence of God and not be bothered by excessive noise.

1–3. Same as 1–3 above.

4. While your friend continues to sit, stand up and lift your arms into the air at about shoulder height, with palms facing the heavens. Visualize three beams of light: One beam of gold/white light comes from the heavens onto the crown of your head (*Keter*), a second beam of gold/white light comes down onto the palm and fingers of the left hand, and a third beam of gold/white light comes down onto the palm and fingers of the right hand. Know with an internal knowledge that the *Sefirot* (which you will visualize in your fingers) are divine energies that allow us to connect the divine part within ourselves to the Divine Ruler of the Universe — this is how the Immanent Feminine merges with the Transcendent Masculine.

5. Feel the beams of light coming down into the palms and fingers of each hand and your *Keter,* crown. Bring Rabbi Hezekiah's prayer of focusing on the number 10 to your awareness. Then say to yourself the name of the energies of each of the ten *Sefirot* and visualize them on your ten fingers (p.149).

6. Now stand behind the individual who is to receive healing, with your left palm and fingers facing the person's left temporal lobe and the right palm and fingers facing his/her right temporal lobe. See/know that the energies of *Bina, Gevurah, Hod, Yesod,* and *Malchut* are flowing through and from your left hand into his/her left temporal lobe, and the energy of *Keter, Chochma, Chesed,*

Tiferet, and *Netzach* are flowing through and from your right hand into his/her right temporal lobe.

7. Breathe in gently and deeply to the count of six, visualizing the beam of light at *Keter,* the crown of your head, flowing into your heart.

8. Hold your breath to the count of three, visualizing *Tiferet,* your heart, filled with light.

9. Breathe out gently through your nostrils to the count of six and see *Tiferet* energy move from your heart across your chest, down both arms, and out of the fingers of your left and right hands. As you breathe out, remember that the left hand has the *Sefirotic* energies of *Bina, Gevurah, Hod, Yesod, and Malchut* and the right hand has the *Sefirotic* energies of *Keter, Chochma, Chesed, Tiferet,* and *Netzach.* The masculine and feminine energies of the right and left fingers are being aligned and balanced through the *Tiferet* energy of the heart. Therefore, visualize every temporal lobe cell in proper balance, receiving *Tiferet* balanced energies of all ten *Sefirot.*

10. Know that the presence and power of God's energy are re-established in every cell of the temporal lobes.

11. Repeat steps 7–10 two more times. At the conclusion of the third time, thank God profusely with sincerity and with love for bringing mental healing to your friend.

12. See your friend well and happy and thank God again for healing your friend.

HOW TO: Eliminate Depression by Freeing the *Shechina* from Her Exile and Reuniting Her with Her Male Consort

1. Both you and your friend should sit facing each other. Hold hands with one another.

2. With your eyes closed, visualize a beam of gold/white light coming down from the heavens onto *Keter* the crown of your head. The light is filled with many purple sets of *YHVH* יהוה.

3. Inhale gently but deeply through your nostrils. As you do, activate the beam of light so that, when you breathe in, it is activated and travels through *Keter* into *Tiferet,* your heart.

4. Hold your breath for 3–4 seconds and see your heart filled with light with many purple sets of *YHVH* יהוה.

5. As you breathe out through your nostrils, silently say, "You shall love the Lord your God with all your heart, with all your soul, with all your might." When you get to the word "heart," visualize your heart opening up, so that the healing light/energy of your heart with the sets of purple YHVH יהוה flows through the air into your friend, filling every single cell of her/his body with purple YHVH יהוה. Feel or intuit every cell in your friend's body — every cell — receiving healing light/energy. View yourself as a vessel of divine healing energy.

6. Continue holding hands with your friend as you sit opposite one another. Again, visualize the beam of light with sets of purple YHVH יהוה coming down from the heavens, onto *Keter*, your crown. Again, gently breathe in through your nostrils and visualize healing light/energy moving down through *Keter* into *Tiferet* your heart area.

7. Hold your breath for 3–4 seconds, and see your heart filled with divine light/energy.

8. As you exhale through your nostrils, say to yourself, "You shall love the Lord your God with all your heart, all your soul and all your might." When you say *heart*, again visualize your heart opening up, but this time visualize the divine light/energy, filled with purple sets of YHVHs יהוה flowing from your heart to specifically the temporal lobes of your friend. The YHVH energies lift up the ADNY אדני energies in your friend's temporal lobe cells, so that the Exile is over. I visualize the ADNY in green. Each cell of your friend's temporal lobes now contain יאהדונהי in joined energies in green and purple. Every cell is healthy and strong.

9. Speak silently while holding hands just as Rabbi Nachman taught: "happy temporal lobe cells (ten times) . . . strong temporal lobe cells (ten times) . . . healthy temporal lobe cells (ten times) . . . balanced and healed temporal lobe cells (ten times). Visualize in your mind's eye יאהדונהי in purple and green in every cell.

10. Thank God for healing your friend of depression and know that a great *teshuvah*, soul restoration, has taken place. Your friend has returned and accepted God with the Greater Mind, and every cell has returned to its original perfect code as it was, יאהדונהי. Thank God.

19

Nekavim, Nekavim, Chalulim, Chalulim

W E understand now that prayer is a means of *connecting*—connecting with the divine in ourselves, connecting the divine in ourselves with the divine in (and beyond) this world, and connecting with the divine in others. The Hebrew word for prayer, *tefila*, also means to connect. It seems appropriate to conclude this phase of our study with a slightly more expanded glimpse into connections that can be made.

Peggy and I hope this slightly broader perspective will inspire you to join us for exploring some of these details even more deeply, in offerings to appear on our Web site (HealingWithGodsLove.com) and in further publications. In this chapter, please be aware that we are using the term "Man" much as we have used the term "God" throughout this book — that is, as inclusive of both genders, and something more of a complex spiritual nature. It is the feminine side that receives while the masculine side delivers. Each has its own place in the Cosmos and each, when coming together in the right way with the right intentionality, allows for the power of prayer to explode.

The *Sefirot* are our source. They are the ten raw materials of the Cosmos. They also are the building blocks of our individual personalities. We humans are the *Sefirot* in action. All things — even every thought, feeling, and word — are made up of the ten *Sefirot*. They form the spiritual DNA pattern underlying everything.

The Hebrew letters are energies created by the interaction of the *Sefirot* at the dawn of Creation. As we've discussed, the *Sefirot* and these twenty-two different energy forms originate from the infinite source of the *Ayn Sof.* The *Sefirot* are holographic — each *Sefira* has ten *Sefirot* within it, *ad infinitum.* So, in reality, the *Sefirot* are infinite in number, not just the ten.

Within the *Sefirotic* Universe, the *Sefirot* are divided into worlds or *olamot.* Each *olam* (world) is not really a physical world, but a realm of *Sefirotic* energy. Each realm is a spiritual level of the universe, allowing us to be aware on different levels of the nature of God.

There are five realms or worlds. Even though we speak of them as first and second and third, there is no temporal priority in their arisal or reality. There is only logical priority. All the worlds are parallel and simultaneous. Each expresses in accordance to the *Sefira* which formed it.

For example, the first world is called *Adam Kadmon* or Primordial Man and is the realm of *Keter.* This *Sefira* is the spark of God from which everything comes into being. One might say that *Adam Kadmon* is the design of everything in creation. Even though all the worlds derive from *Adam Kadmon,* this realm itself cannot be understood or revealed. That's why when we refer to the worlds of the universe, we don't actually count *Adam Kadmon.* We only count the next four.

The highest world to manifest is the "second" world in the lesser known schema of five worlds, and at the same time the "first world" in the familiar schema of four worlds. It is known as *Atzilut,* which means Emanation. We know that this realm is closest to the divine Source or *Adam Kadmon.* In *Atzilut,* we simply cannot discern *Adam Kadmon* as a separate identity. There is no manifestation of diversity at all in *Atzilut.* It is like the Tree of Life in which all is One. It is the realm of Pure Spirit, Divine Will — the exclusive realm of God. While this world is beyond human comprehension, we do know that its light descends into the lower worlds. The dominant *Sefira* of *Atzilut* is *Chochma.*

The world below this is called *Briah,* the world of Creation. It is the world of Mind, and also of souls. These souls are spoken of as the throne of God. God not only dwells within them, but upon them. *Briah* is the source of Judgment in the world. Here we can first discern separate identity, even though it is highly spiritualized. *Bina* is the dominant *Sefira* here.

The next world, in logical priority, is the world of *Yetzirah,* the realm of Emotion. The *Yetziratic* entities are not souls, as in *Briah,* but angels. The word *Yetzirah* means Formation. *Yetzirah* gave and gives form to time, so is considered the realm of Time. In this world the six *Sefirot* below *Bina*, collectively called the *Middot*, are dominant.

The world in which we live physically is called *Assiyah* and corresponds to the *Sefira Malchut*. It is the realm of Matter, the corporeal.

The four worlds are abbreviated as אבי״ע. Since the Kabbalah is holographic, each world has a complete אבי״ע within it. They are also divine energy levels, such as spiritual energies of the angelic world, thought-energies of the soul world, and so on. When we discuss a world, we also want to know what level within the realm we are discussing.

In *Atzilut*, God's unity is recognized in all. We don't see God's unity as clearly in the worlds of *Briah, Yetzirah,* and *Assiyah.* The human mind has two functions: to experience the conscious world and to experience the unconscious. Pure thought originates in the world of *Briah*, Mind, whereas emotion originates in *Yetzirah.* We experience *Yetziratic* reality in our unconscious mind. We experience the world of *Briah* through our conscious mind.

It is fascinating that renowned physicists such as Stephen Hawking recognize that our universe or world isn't the only universe and say, similar to Kabbalah, that there are universes parallel to ours. Hawking maintains that a version of each of us exists in each of these parallel universes.

This means that if someone is ill in this physical world, he/she has to have a healthy parallel in another universe. If we could find the code for the parallel universe where the healthy person lives, we would be able to effect great healing. But wait — we do have these codes! They aren't being held in scientific vaults, they are in Kabbalistic treatises on prayer. Each of these codes allows us to connect the divine part within ourselves with the corresponding aspect of the Divine that governs the universe.

This is exactly what we do when we pray for the well-being of others. We draw down the transcendent light of *YHVH* יהוה and at the same time lift up the *Shechina* light of *Adonai* אד״נ. When we pray this way, we become vessels for healing.

We learn in our Talmud about Rabbi Nehunia ben HaKanah who was a *baal shem tov*, a master of prayer. A *baal shem tov* is a person who knows what energies to use when praying for the sick. But Rabbi Nehunia transcended even that knowledge. He not only would pray for the sick, he actually would know whether his prayers were answered, or had connected. He knew about the parallel worlds. When he prayed for someone who was sick, he visualized these worlds, and if he saw a world in which the person was healed, he knew his prayers were answered.

One who can pray with the understanding of the Four (or Five) Worlds can perceive the Tree of Life reality — where everything is connected and all is One — as distinct from the Tree of Knowledge reality where diversity, plurality, and duality operate. The master of prayer visualizes a Tree of Life world, a world of *Atzilut*, and sees a vast quantum web of connection where parts of one thing and parts of another thing continuously trade places. The master of prayer sees the world's operations not through the activity of individual things, but in the connections between them and in the space between them. In this space, he/she sees healing and brings it, through prayer, into this world of *Assiyah*.

Rabbi Nehunia ben HaKanah was able to see, in a higher world, a situation of this world before something caused a disruption in the person's spiritual DNA. He was able to see the sick person's cells as in an undifferentiated state and, through visualization and prayer, bring healing to that person from God. Remember: Kabbalah teaches us that God created healing even before He created this world. This healing is stored in the celestial worlds, and through unique mystical prayers we can bring healing "down" into this world.

Man (and Woman) is the goal of God's creation. All the spiritual worlds exist for our sake in that God created the universe in such a way that it remains incomplete unless we fulfill our purpose, which is to realize God's plan. God created *Atzilut, Briah, Yetzirah,* and *Assiyah* as distinct from one another, and created Man to join all of them together.

Here is a wonderful meditation on how to travel in the various worlds.

HOW TO: Meditation on the Four Worlds as Taught by the Baal Shem Tov

1. Sit in a quiet place, your *mi'at meekdash*.
2. Be aware of your breathing. Breathe quietly and deeply.

3. Think of the activities you plan to do later in the day. Think of the people you will meet, the work you will do. All this belongs to the world of *Assiyah*. Know that this is God's light in the physical world.

4. Continue to breathe in and out and visualize your interactions with different people during the day. See yourself talking and speaking with them and know that all this speech-energy is part of the Speech world of *Yetzirah*. See the light of God pervading these conversations and think of God within the realm of *Yetzirah*. Continue breathing quietly and deeply.

5. Now focus on your inner thought process. See how your thought process affects your emotions. As you do this, you are in the world of *Briah*, the world of Soul.

6. Breathe deeply and gently and recognize that behind everything there is life. As you recognize this, you become aware in the world of *Atzilut*, where everything that previously seemed disparate and separate is really connected by the Spirit of God. This is the case whether it be your computer or your boss, or your pet dog — within them all is the Soul of God. This is the world of *Atzilut*.

Asher Yatzar Prayer:
The Great Healing Prayer of the Body

In the early 1990s, I met someone who has become a good friend — Armando Rivera, our synagogue custodian. Armando not only has been responsible for the well-being of our synagogue, but for many years also attended to the well-being of our dogs. He walked them every day and they loved him, as did we. One day, about twelve years ago, as he and I were both leaving the bathroom, Armando told me, "When I go the bathroom, I always say a prayer to God thanking Him that everything is working."

Armando didn't realize at the time how profound his insight was. Jewish tradition mandates that the observant Jew say the *Asher Yatzar* prayer every morning to thank God that, indeed, "everything is working." With its knowledge and acknowledgment of our bodily functions, this prayer has a profound impact on healing.

בָּרוּךְ אַתָּה, יְיָ אֱלֹהֵינוּ, מֶלֶךְ הָעוֹלָם,

אֲשֶׁר יָצַר אֶת הָאָדָם בְּחָכְמָה,

וּבָרָא בוֹ נְקָבִים נְקָבִים, חֲלוּלִים חֲלוּלִים.

גָּלוּי וְיָדוּעַ לִפְנֵי כִסֵּא כְבוֹדֶךָ,

שֶׁאִם יִפָּתֵחַ אֶחָד מֵהֶם, אוֹ יִסָּתֵם אֶחָד מֵהֶם,

אִי אֶפְשָׁר לְהִתְקַיֵּים וְלַעֲמוֹד לְפָנֶיךָ.

בָּרוּךְ אַתָּה יְיָ, רוֹפֵא כָל בָּשָׂר וּמַפְלִיא לַעֲשׂוֹת.

Baruch atah Adonai eloheinu melech ha'olam asher yatzar et ha'adam b'chochmah u'vara vo n'kavim n'kavim chalulim chalulim. Galu'i v'yadua lifnei kisei k'vodecha she'im yipatei'ach echad me'hem o yisataim echad me'hem ee efshar l'hitkayeim v'la'amod lefanecha afilu sha'ah achat. Baruch atah Adonai rofeh chol basar u'mafli la'asot.

Praised are You, O Lord our God, King of the Universe, who has formed man with wisdom and created within him, nekavim, nekavim, chalulim, chalulim. It is revealed and known before the seat of Your honor that if one of these be opened, or one of these be closed, it would be impossible to survive and stand before You, even for a moment. Praised are You O Lord, Healer of all flesh and worker of wonders.

In this blessing written centuries ago, the liturgical author praises *Hashem*. He states that the Lord *Hashem* is clearly continuously involved in keeping us alive, creating and sustaining within us *nekavim, nekavim* — many openings, and *chalulim, chalulim* — many hollow spaces. Without God's Presence working within us continuously, we would not be able to survive for a single moment. The author of the prayer thanks *Hashem* for creating systems of nerves, arteries, veins, and blood vessels that supply all 248 organs — our *chalulim* — with different energies and nutrients, and a system of digestion that absorbs the nutrients and eliminates waste, *nekavim, nekavim*. If even a single organ is injured greatly and if even one container be blocked, we could not survive. "Praised are You, O Lord, Healer of all flesh and worker of wonders."

The *Asher Yatzar* blessing is near the beginning of our Jewish prayer book, liberal or Orthodox. It is to be recited every morning as part of the morning blessings, *Birkat HaShachar,* recognizing that God is the Great Healer. After saying the *Modeh Ani* prayer, thanking *Hashem* for restoring one's soul, one goes to the bathroom, relieves oneself, and thanks God for the wondrous working of one's body. We see in this blessing that our bodies are complex systems and how, if one part fails, that affects our whole body. When we recite this blessing, we need to recognize that, as we pray, God is doing the healing. We need to say this blessing in the Greater Mind.

It is fascinating that our rabbis wrote this blessing more than two thousand years ago. Within the first two pages of the prayer book, we recognize the holistic nature of our faith, and that God and man work together in prayer to maintain a living soul and a living body.

"Man" is the Healing Conduit between God and Creation

The *Asher Yatzar* is my single favorite prayer because in it we see the holistic nature of Kabbalistic healing. Not only are we mandated to say it every morning after we go to the bathroom and wash our hands, observant Jews are obligated to say it every time we use the washroom throughout the day. I believe it is extremely important to use this *brucha* (blessing) every time we need healing. As we will see, it not only brings healing to the person who prays or receives the blessing of these sacred energies. It also has the power to heal the cosmos.

The medieval Kabbalist Rabbi Maier Ibn Gabbei taught that God formed Man in such a way that all the revealed and hidden universes are included within Man in exact miniature. We know that the Kabbalah speaks of five supernal universes, but a secret of Kabbalistic teaching is that each of these universes is called Adam or Man as well. In descending order of magnitude, there is *Adam Kadmon,* the universe of Primordial Man; then *Adam d'Atzilut,* universe of Emanation; then *Adam d'Briah,* universe of Creation; then *Adam d'Yetzirah,* universe of Formation. Finally there is *Adam d'Assiyah,* the universe of Action, our physical world.

The rabbis are teaching that the human body is created in the image of God, according to the blueprint of this great system of universes. Just as each limb, organ, and sinew in the human body is part of a unified organism, so every universe and all the universes form one complete unified structure. Everything is connected with everything and creation is governed by God, who is within every universe as well as within every single organ and limb of Man. In this teaching, Man becomes the *animating soul* of all the universes. With aspects of all the worlds within him, he is the blueprint of *Atzilut, Briah, Yetzirah,* and *Assiyah* and the connecting link God created to join them as One.

This is what makes the *Asher Yatzar* so powerful as a healing prayer. As the Animating Soul of the universe, Man is in a unique position to bring down to this world of *Assiyah* the healing secrets of the supernal worlds. Man is the *raison d'être* for the creation of all the worlds, so he can deliver great healing to the Cosmos. When one prays the *Asher Yatzar* healing blessing, with this mindset, it has enormous healing power.

Man is in a constant state of flux, as his life force and attention and awareness travel spiritually through different universes. This spiritual movement greatly affects the physical, spiritual, and Godly realms of the entire cosmos — through individual expressions of aspiration, thoughts, and deeds, combined with individual awareness of the unity of God. This secret allows us to understand that "healing" is given to Man as co-partner with God. God is the Great Healer, and Man is the instrument through which He heals.

Rabbi Chaim of Volozhin teaches that "God created Man in His Image" means that Man, with his divine soul, controls all spiritual influence and manifestation. The ancient rabbis who created the *Asher Yatzar* understood clearly that this healing prayer is not only about Man's physical arterial functioning, it is also about the connection of the multiple worlds invested in Man's creation. Because Man's soul is rooted in the world of *Atzilut,*

Man has access to the highest manifestations of the Infinite and is able to draw them into this world as spiritual and physical healing. Man thus becomes a bridge between the supernal and lower worlds, exactly as God intended. Man is the healing conduit between God and creation.

All the universes are the Name of God, in its various degrees of revelation:

Adam Kadmon apex

י   *Atzilut*

ה   *Briah*

ו   *Yetzirah*

ה   *Assiyah*

Man's mission is to reveal *Atzilut*, the world of Emanation. This gets accomplished in our lower world of *Assiyah* through healing prayer. Man's unique connection to God contains the potential to reveal God within the physical. Spanning the universes, Man combines the infinite with the finite as his soul travels throughout the supernal worlds. This soul has the ability to reveal the Presence of God through focused meditative practice and healing prayer, drawing divine energies into corporeal reality.

At that Thanksgiving dinner Peggy and I enjoyed with minister friends — where we discussed "love" in the Hebrew and Christian scriptures — we also discussed this idea. One of the ministers (actually he was a student minister at the time) asked me, "When, in the early pages of Genesis, God says, 'Let Us make Man in our image,' isn't He referring to Jesus? Who else would God be talking to, Douglas?"

I said that God could be talking to the angels. As a matter of fact, I mentioned, there is a Jewish Midrash that teaches that the angels warned God not to create Man, lest there be bloodshed.

As the Hebrew letters have souls, each being a unique energetic force, it's likely God consulted with them, too, when He created the universes. We learn in our Kabbalah that God spoke to all the universes, "Let Us make Man in Our Image." *Briah* was destined to give Man that aspect of soul called *Neshamah*, or divine breath. *Yetzirah* would give Man his *Ru'ach* or spirit. *Assiyah* would give him his *Nefesh* soul. Then *Hashem* gave Man from *Atzilut* a living soul, "He breathed into his nostrils a living soul."

From this we learn that when we pray this prayer with *kavvanah*, when we pray the *Asher Yatzar* with the Greater Mind, not only do we activate the Presence of God — so that every vessel, every orifice, every organ, every limb work wonderfully well — but we bind all the universes together.

This prayer has celestial and cosmic purpose and power. It brings great healing not only in the bathroom but also in the hospital room, the bedroom, the sanctuary of the synagogue, and even in the cosmos. It is a wonderful instrument of healing. I often use this healing prayer, and teach others how to use it, after surgery or during illness.

Philologically, the words *nekavim, nekavim* and *chalulim, chalulim*, translate as "many openings" and "many hollow spaces," respectively. But the ancient writer of this blessing does not offer only a philological insight. He also, when repeating the words, offers us a kind of poetry in motion about the dual nature of being Man. On one side is our human nature, within which God created a complex and sophisticated system of channels and passageways and organs and limbs. On the other side, Man is not only a complex body of organs, but is a highly spiritual being. "He" is the *Nefesh Chayah,* or the Animating Soul of all the universes. All the universes were created as instruments through which we can draw close to God. According to Rabbi Moses Cordovero, the universes are filters that allow us to draw near to God and at the same time not be obliterated by His light.

Nekavim, Nekavim, Chalulim, Chalulim

Each of us can draw upon this teaching of Man as the *Nefesh Chayah,* the Animating Soul of all the universes, whose life force affects everything in them. The power of this *brucha* is amazing. When we pray the right words with the proper intent, there is healing in the cosmos and in the human body.

A healing meditation that I suggest for use while recuperating from surgery is to say again and again as a mantra — *nekavim, nekavim, chalulim, chalulim* — at least twenty-six times. As you say this powerful Hebrew phrase, know that God is healing you from head to toe, whether you had heart surgery, kidney surgery, skin surgery, or any other kind. Visualize yourself well, with the knowledge that God is healing you. While thinking this, say: *nekavim, nekavim, chalulim, chalulim,* acknowledging that God is healing your body completely. Recognize that your soul is so loved by God that She is animating all the beings and all the universes, drawing you closer and closer to healing angels, who are pouring out God's healing prayers on your behalf.

As you recite this Hebrew phrase, you are recognizing your dual nature. You are a man or woman, created with a complex system of orifices and organs. At the same time, you are a soul that has the power to inspire the angels and all the celestial worlds of God's creation to bring about healing.

People who are comfortable with Hebrew, or who will become more comfortable with Hebrew through practice, can say this blessing with even greater voltage. I suggest strongly that when you have the flu, or are about to enter surgery, or if you have just experienced surgery, you use this blessing as an adjunct to the many healing meditative practices offered in this book.

HOW TO: Use *Asher Yatzar* Healing Blessing with Increased Voltage, before or after Surgery

1. Sit or lie down, either in your hospital bed or your *mi'at meekdash.* Make yourself comfortable and be conscious of your breathing. Recognize that you have within you a sacred soul, a *Nefesh Chayah,* that regulates not only the workings of your body, but the workings of the cosmos. Recognize the dual nature of being a person.

2. Repeat as a mantra, *nekavim, nekavim, chalulim, chalulim* twenty-six times. (26 is equal to the *gematria* of *YHVH.*) Recite the *Asher Yatzar* blessing in Hebrew or in English, as found above on page 254. As you are reciting this blessing, recognize through *Mohin de Gadlut* that *Hashem* is healing all your passageways, hollow ways, and organs. He will guide your surgeon meticulously well, to the extent that when surgery is over, you will be well.

3. Say the *Asher Yatzar* blessing one more time, with *Mohin de Gadlut.*

4. See yourself completely well after the surgery. Thank God for having healed you.

It may be difficult to say this blessing immediately after surgery, but when you are awake and clear minded, perhaps after several days, do it as outlined above.

One can do the *Asher Yatzar* prayer as a blessing for another person. Remember, a prayer is when you pray for yourself; a blessing is when you pray for another person.

HOW TO: Use the *Asher Yatzar* Healing Prayer for Another Person

This prayer can be said both before and after surgery.

1. Sit next to the person you are praying for, and recognize that *Hashem* is right there with you both.

2. Repeat silently as a mantra *nekavim, nekavim, chalulim, chalulim* twenty-six times (counting on your fingers). While you are doing this meditation, know that you are an instrument of God.

3. Hold hands with the person you are praying for, and recite the healing prayer of *Asher Yatzar* three times. Do this with the conviction that *Hashem* is animating and enlivening every limb, every organ, every channel of your friend's body. Know with certainty that *Hashem* is using you as a *Nefesh Chayah,* an Animating Soul, to heal your friend's illness. As you recite this prayer three times, visualize all his/her organs working well with one another — digestive system, circulatory system, nervous system, etc., all working in harmony. Know that *Hashem*, through you, is healing your friend. Visualize the doctors doing a wonderful job. See your friend well and healed.

4. Thank God for healing your friend.

Epilogue

I T IS VERY IMPORTANT to recognize that God is within each one of us, occupying every cell and every soul of each one of us. Rabbi Nachman of Breslov has had the greatest effect on me and my desire to be with God, work with God, love God, and play with God on an ongoing basis. It is Rabbi Nachman who, among others, teaches that the divine split that took place in the Garden of Eden was the beginning of a new friendship between Man (and Woman) and God. God felt such empathy for us when *Hashem* exiled us from the glorious Garden that She went into exile with us and within us.

Each day we need to focus on the different meditative practices that show us how God, the Feminine, and God, the Masculine, have the potential to be One — if we, because of our love for Her, can focus on the *kavvanot* that show us that God not only is One, but is One in all of us. She manifests Her Feminine Nature and He manifests His Masculine Nature through us, through *Ribbono shel Olam*'s love for us. The *Shechina* eagerly waits to be liberated from Her imprisonment and join in joy with *Hashem*'s Masculine Presence, then balance takes place and amazing joyous healing follows.

We do not repair a split God through meditation mantras alone. The most important thing I can emphasize for you to do is to live an ethical life. Every day, be as kind as you can to your fellow human beings, little animals, and our planet. This gives God strength.

We also firmly believe in the power of twenty-first-century medicine — Western and alternative — and see how this power can be joined with the equal power of Kabbalistic teachings. We need to do this through *Mohin de Gadlut,* the Greater Mind, where fear plays no part.

God wants you to call upon Him, so His abundance can fill your every cell and every soul. And with God, all things are possible. We are His children. He loves us. We love Him. *Baruch Hashem.*

I would love to hear how you are doing as you practice these different *kavvanot.* You can contact me through our Web site HealingwithGodsLove. com. As the site develops, you also can see video demonstrations of some of the meditations and listen to audios intended to help you master some of the Hebrew words. You'll also see a selection of my paintings, of which one is featured on the front cover of this book, and eight are rendered in black and white inside.

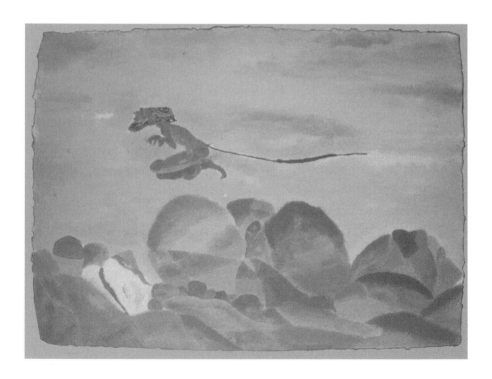

The *Sh'ma* Meditation and the *Sefirot*

The *Sh'ma* prayer consists of three paragraphs. The first and second lines which we commonly know as the *Sh'ma* prayer — *Sh'ma Yis'ra'el, YHVH Eloheinu YHVH Echad. Baruch shem k'vod Malchuto l'olam va'ed; Hear O Israel, YHVH is our God, YHVH is One* — are part of the first paragraph. The sources of the first two paragraphs are Deuteronomy 6:4–9 and Deuteronomy 11:13–21. The third paragraph is Numbers 15:37–41. These three paragraphs, plus the first three words of the next prayer: *YHVH Eloheihem Emet* — *YHVH, Our God is Truth* — add up to 248 words, which is equal to the number of limbs and organs in the human body. From this we discover that there is a connection between the physical body, the recitation of the *Sh'ma,* and healing.

The Hebrew language has twenty-two consonant letters. It also has vowel marks distinct from the letters. The ancient Kabbalah correlates these vowel marks with different *Sefirot*, or transformers of Divine energy located in

Sefira	Vowel			Tetragrammaton	
Keter	Kametz	a	אָ	YaHaVaHa	יְהֹוָה
Chochma	Patach	a	אַ	YaHaVaHa	יֲהֲוֲה
Bina	Tzeré	e	אֵ	YeHeVeHe	יֵהֵוֵה
Chesed	Segol	e	אֶ	YeHeVeHe	יֶהֶוֶה
Gevurah	Sh'va	'	אְ	Y'H'V'H'	יְהְוְה
Tiferet	Cholem	o	אֹ	YoHoVoHo	יֹהֹוֹה
Netzach	Chirek	i	אִ	YiHiViHi	יִהִוִה
Hod	Kibbutz	u	אֻ	YuHuVuHu	יֻהֻוֻה
Yesod	Shurek	u	אוּ	YuHuVuHu	יוּהוּוּה
Malchut	no vowel			YHVH	יהוה

different parts of the human body. When we do Kabbalistic healing, we need to align the *Sefirotic* Tree with our body.

When we look at the human body and the placement of the *Sefirot* on the body, we need to remember that this arrangement is based on the picture of the original Cosmic Man, God's original blueprint with which He created Man and Woman. Every vowel mark correlates with a different *Sefira* on this cosmic map of Man and on the human body of each of us.

The first two sentences of the *Sh'ma* contain all these *Sefirot*. Therefore when we recite the first and second lines of the *Sh'ma* prayer, we are connected with God's Divine Light in every part of our body.

שְׁמַע יִשְׂרָאֵל יהוה אֱלֹהֵינוּ יהוה אֶחָד

בָּרוּךְ שֵׁם כְּבוֹד מַלְכוּתוֹ לְעוֹלָם וָעֶד

Sh'ma Yis'ra'el YHVH El o hei nu YHVH E chad.
Baruch Shem K'vod Malchuto L'olam Va'ed.

In the Hebrew line above, **starting at the right,** you see the first syllable שְׁ *Sh*, is vocalized with a *sh'va* :, two dots, one above the other. It represents the *Sefira Gevurah,* which communicates the energy of strength or restraint.

The second syllable, מַע *ma*, is vocalized with the *patach* – , a horizontal straight line. It represents *Chochma*, which communicates the energy of wisdom, or intuitive knowledge.

The next syllable יִשְׂ *Yis*, is vocalized with the *chirek* •, a single dot. It represents *Netzach*, which communicates the energy of Eternity or Victory.

The next syllable רָ *ra*, is vocalized with the *kametz* ⊤, two intersecting lines. It represents *Keter*, or Crown, which communicates God's Divine Energy.

The next syllable in the prayer אֵל *el*, is vocalized with a *tzere* ••, two dots side by side. It represents *Bina*, which communicates the energy of rational thought.

YHVH יהוה has no vowels, and is related to *Malchut*, the Feminine Presence of God, or Kingdom, within us.

The next syllable we see is אֶל *El*.[1] It is vocalized with a *segol* •••, three dots in a triangle. It represents *Chesed*, which communicates the energy of Compassion.

The next syllable *o*, is vocalized with the *cholem* וֹ, a vertical line with a dot on top. It represents *Tiferet*, which communicates the energy of Balance or Harmony.

We then come to the syllable הֵי *hei*, vocalized with the *tzere* ••, representing *Bina*, which communicates the energy of Rational Knowledge.

The next syllable נוּ *nu*, is vocalized with a vertical line or *vav* beside a middle dot the *shurek* וּ. It represents *Yesod*, which communicates Foundational Energy.

The *YHVH* יהוה again is *Malchut*, with no vowels.

The syllable אֶ *E* is vocalized with the *segol* ••, representing *Chesed*, which communicates Compassionate energy.

And חָד *chad* is vocalized with the *kametz* ָ, representing *Keter*, the Divine Source.

Reading Hebrew right to left	Reading transliteration left to right	Sefirot	Body part	English
שְׁ מַ ע	Sh ma	Gevurah Chochma	left shoulder right brain	*Hear*
יִשְׂ רָ אֵל	Yis ra el,	Netzach Keter Bina	right hip crown of head left brain	*O Israel,*
יהוה	YHVH	Malchut	coccyx, feet	*YHVH*
אֱלֹ הֵי נוּ	El o hei nu,	Chesed Tiferet Bina Yesod	right shoulder chest left brain lower abdomen	*is our God*
יהוה	YHVH	Malchut	coccyx, feet	*YHVH*
אֶ חָד	E chad.	Chesed Keter	right shoulder crown of head	*is One.*

Thus, the first line of the *Sh'ma* represents nine *Sefirot*. The second line, *Baruch Shem K'vod Malchuto L'olam Va'ed*, symbolizes the *Sefira Hod*, for the total of ten *Sefirot*. It is related to the Hebrew word *Hodu*, which means "giving thanks." *Hod*, the *Sefira*, represents the Energy of Humility; the humble person always gives thanks. So the second line of the *Sh'ma* recognizes God's Kingdom with thanks and humility, communicating the *Sefira* of *Hod*.

A Kabbalistic Healing Meditation

שְׁמַע יִשְׂרָאֵל יהוה אֱלֹהֵינוּ יהוה אֶחָד

Sh'ma Yis'ra'el YHVH El o hei nu YHVH E chad.
Hear O Israel, YHVH is our God, YHVH is One.

Rabbi Nachman of Breslov teaches that the *Sh'ma* draws joy and healing into all of our 248 limbs and organs. Here is one of his healing meditations based on the *Sh'ma*. Rabbi Nachman of Breslov teaches that the *Sh'ma* draws joy and healing into all of our 248 limbs and organs. Here is one of his healing meditations based on the *Sh'ma*.

As you sit relaxed, recite the *Sh'ma* prayer very slowly, syllable by syllable, recognizing that the energy of *Ayn Sof*, the Infinite, is in the air and, through your built-in transformers of *Ayn Sof*'s Divine Energy, or *Sefirot*, you are bringing healing to all your limbs and organs.

Slowly recite the *Sh'ma*, identifying each vowel with a different energy center of the Divine: *Sh' Ma Yis Ra El* . . . As you recite the *Sh'ma*, look at the diagram above, knowing that, as you do this, the *Sh'ma* itself sends God's healing energy to the 248 limbs and organs of your body.

As you are saying the *Sh'ma*, you are visualizing and feeling God's Divine Energy being transformed by each of the *Sefirot*. Remember the second line of the *Sh'ma* communicates the Divine energy of *Hod*:

בָּרוּךְ שֵׁם כְּבוֹד מַלְכוּתוֹ לְעוֹלָם וָעֶד

Baruch Shem K'vod Malchuto L'olam Va'ed.
Blessed be the Name of His glorious kingdom for ever and ever.

The *Sh'ma* prayer testifies to the ten aspects of Divine Energy manifesting in your body, bringing about wonderful healing.

Ayin is the last letter of the word *Sh'ma*. *Daled* is the last letter of the word *Echad*. Together, *Ayin Daled* means witness: "You are a witness to your own healing." When you put the letters together backwards, it becomes *da*, to know. So, it says, know that you are a witness. The word *da* is hidden in the *Sh'ma* prayer. It is a Kabbalistic secret that witnesses to the tremendous healing power of the *Sh'ma* prayer.

NOTE

1. The point we're focusing on here is the relationship between *Chesed* and the *segol*. So don't be confused or distracted by seeing five dots here instead of only three. Hebrew grammar requires some guttural letters, such as *Alef* in this case, to have a composite *sh'va* (one dot on top of another), to get strength to the *segol*. That's why you see five dots under the *Alef* here, but what matters in our present context is only the *segol*.

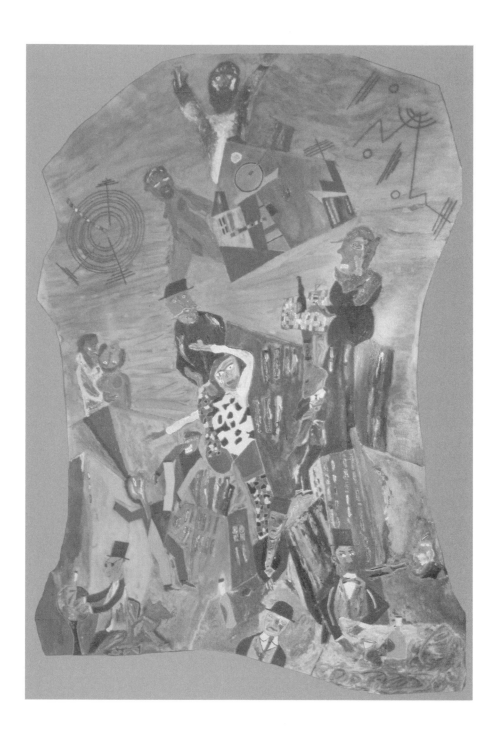

Index